The Successful Chinese Herbalist

Bob Flaws and Honora Lee Wolfe

2005
Blue Poppy Press

Published by:
BLUE POPPY PRESS
A Division of Blue Poppy Enterprises, Inc.
1990 North 57th Court, Unit A
BOULDER, CO 80301

First Edition, May 2005
Second Printing, August 2010

ISBN 978-1-891845-29-2
LCCN #2005923635

10 9 8 7 6 5 4 3 2

Printed at Edwards Brothers, Ann Arbor, MI
on acid-free paper and soy inks

Text and cover design by Eric J. Brearton

Table of Contents

PREFACE . . . .   **v**

CHAPTER 1. The Importance of Pattern Discrimination
in Crafting the Best Formula **1**

CHAPTER 2. Writing a Formula That Works for
Each Patient **27**

CHAPTER 3. Forms of Chinese Herbal Medicines & Their
Appropriate Use **63**

CHAPTER 4. Potency Issues with Chinese Herbal
Medicine **71**

CHAPTER 5. The Issue of Dose in Ready-made
Medicines **79**

CHAPTER 6. The Phenomenon of Habituation in Long-term
Herbal Treatment **87**

CHAPTER 7. Possible Problems with Ready-made
Medicines **93**

CHAPTER 8. The Three Important Types of Potential
Medicinal Toxicity **99**

CHAPTER 9. Using Chinese Herbs During Pregnancy and
Lactation **107**

CHAPTER 10. My Favorite Formulas **113**

CHAPTER 11. How to Set Up & Run an Effective Chinese
Herbal Pharmacy **141**

CHAPTER 12. How to Work with Patients Who Are Taking
Western Medication **157**

APPENDIX I: What's Wrong with the Term "Patent
Medicines?" **163**

APPENDIX II: List of the Most Common Treatment
Principles **169**

APPENDIX III: Patient Herb Instruction Form **177**

APPENDIX IV: Problem Based Learning Exercise
Answers **181**

APPENDIX V: A Representative List of Pesticides and
Heavy Metals Tested by Western Companies
Producing Ready-made
Herbal Medicines **205**

Preface

Several years ago we published a book titled *How to Write a TCM Herbal Formula*. This little volume was, for a time, popular with schools and developed a small but loyal following. However, because the information it presented was limited to the administration of Chinese herbal medicine in decoction, and because it was really only an extra-long essay, at some point it needed to either be revised or to go out of print. Since its sales had never been huge, we allowed the book a quiet demise and transplanted the most important information it contained into other texts. In some senses, this new book is a direct lineal descendant of that first modest, but useful essay, now expanded to include a much broader range of subjects.

There is so much to learn about the practice of any medicine. Some of the more practical elements of day-to-day practice and solutions to some of the more thorny problems that are inevitable can only be learned with time. Still, it is the job of any good teacher to shorten the journey of his or her students by sharing what they have learned by traversing a longer route. Thus, we have, with the publication of this new book, tried to address a variety of issues that are, for a variety of reasons, not always able to be taught in the context of the school clinic.

We have written about our experience both as practitioners and as business people because we feel that the owning and operating of a dispensary is an integral part of the practice of Chinese herbal medicine in the U.S. and other countries where these medicines are not sold in standard pharmacies.

This book is not a materia medica or a formulary text. However, while limited to the practice of Chinese herbal medicine, the scope of the book is fairly broad. It includes discussions about everything we could think of that can and will make a positive difference in any practitioner's level of success. Notably, the information about how to determine dosages using any and all types of Chinese medicines has not previously appeared in the English language literature in this depth. Another chapter discusses the phenomenon of habituation, which is well known in the world of Western medicine but is rarely if ever discussed in Chinese herbal medicine texts.

There is also a small but, we believe, useful chapter about working with patients who are taking Western drugs. Although the information presented here is by no means meant to be definitive and while we are working on a lengthy book on this same subject to be released in 2006, this chapter gives any practitioner a methodology to help them determine the impact of any Western drug on their patient's health and how their treatments, herbal or otherwise, might improve such patient's situation.

Another important feature of this book from our point of view and one that we plan to include in most of our future publications is the problem-based learning exercises. These include case studies and questions at the end of most chapters. There is an answer key for these questions at the end of the book. While it may seem that this feature is mostly added for the sake of students, we have done our best to make the information and questions equally relevant for practitioners.

We feel we must say something here about the first chapter of the book, which is a lengthy exposition on pattern discrimination and the processes one uses with each and every patient in the practice of Chinese herbal medicine. This includes both diagnostic and prescriptive processes. Advanced students and some practitioners may feel this information is unnecessarily emphasized or overly drawn out. Perhaps. However, as we always tell both our under-graduate and post-graduate students, mastery is always mas-tery of the basics, no matter what profession one is practic-ing. And, as teachers working with students all over the U.S. and Western Europe, we find repeatedly that the problems practitioners have with prescribing Chinese herbal medicine are most often due to a breakdown in understanding some part or piece of this process. We want to be absolutely cer-tain that readers at all levels of experience understand how and why the successful prescription of Chinese herbal medi-cine is based on this very clear, logical, and specific process. For those of you who feel this information is already well digested, we beg your indulgence. And who knows, even for the seasoned practitioner, there may be a new kernal of truth that is useful.

Finally, we must say a word about terminology. As in most Blue Poppy books, we have mainly used *A Practical Dictionary of Chinese Medicine* by Nigel Wiseman and Feng Ye as our standard for technical words with clinical implica-tions. While attempting to make the book as accessible and friendly a read as possible, our support of this terminology is based on its precision relative to the Chinese language from which our medicine springs and the fact that any given word can, using this text, be traced back to its Chinese char-acter and all the clinical implications of that character. There simply is no other English language glossary that offers us such precision.

We hope that readers, whether students, new practitioners or seasoned professionals, find this book a welcome addition to their herbal medicine library. As always, we welcome your suggestions on how we might improve our efforts when the time comes for a reprint of this book. It is our desire, with this and every book we publish, to help all students and practitioners of this medicine to be more effective clinically, more successful financially, and more satisfied personally.

Thanks for reading,

Honora Lee Wolfe
Bob Flaws
March 2005

CHAPTER **1**

The Importance of Pattern Discrimination in Crafting the Best Formula

The origins of Chinese herbal medicine

Standard professional Chinese medicine, or what is often called Traditional Chinese Medicine (TCM) in the West, is a specific style of Chinese medicine. Although standard professional Chinese medicine has its roots in the Warring States, Qin, and Han dynasties, as a self-conscious style it was created in the People's Republic of China during the 50s, 60s, and 70s. While this last fact has produced some detractors who believe its origins to be 20th century Communist materialism, modern professional Chinese medicine actually incorporates all of the best of both professional and folk medicine surviving in China from its beginnings. In terms of theory, however, it is primarily based on the highly literate and rational approach to medicine of the *ru yi* or Confucian scholar-doctors going back to the Han dynasty but whose writings became preeminent in later dynasties. These scholar-doctors were, by and large, *fang ji jia* or herbal practitioners and the administration of internal herbal medicinals was their main modality. Thus, modern professional Chinese medicine's defining methodology was developed specifically for the practice of herbal medicine.

According to Chinese texts, the defining methodology of standard professional Chinese medicine as a specific style of Chinese medicine can be summed up in the words *bian zheng lun zhi*. This means basing treatment primarily on the discrimination of patterns.

Understanding patterns & diseases

The first chapter of this book is a treatise on the process of pattern discrimination and the logical procedure we follow with each patient in order to arrive at the correct Chinese herbal formula and treatment plan. For some readers this information may be a review. However, we include this somewhat lengthy exposition because it is the foundation upon which good Chinese herbal medicine is always based. Also, as teachers interacting with students all over the U.S. and Western Europe, we find repeatedly that the problems students and practitioners have with prescribing Chinese herbal medicine are not necessarily because they do not know their herbs or formulas, but more often due to a breakdown of

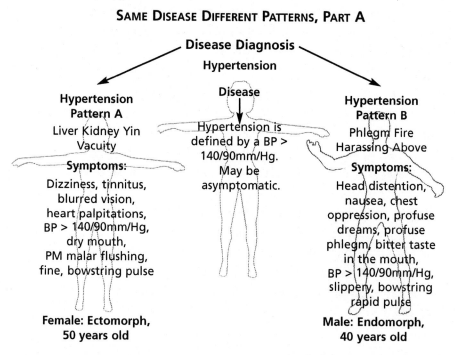

SAME DISEASE DIFFERENT PATTERNS, PART A

Disease Diagnosis

Hypertension

Disease

Hypertension is defined by a BP > 140/90mm/Hg. May be asymptomatic.

Hypertension Pattern A

Liver Kidney Yin Vacuity

Symptoms:

Dizziness, tinnitus, blurred vision, heart palpitations, BP > 140/90mm/Hg, dry mouth, PM malar flushing, fine, bowstring pulse

Female: Ectomorph, 50 years old

Hypertension Pattern B

Phlegm Fire Harassing Above

Symptoms:

Head distention, nausea, chest oppression, profuse dreams, profuse phlegm, bitter taste in the mouth, BP > 140/90mm/Hg, slippery, bowstring rapid pulse

Male: Endomorph, 40 years old

understanding somewhere in this process. Thus, we present as clear an explanation of the process of diagnosis and treatment as we can, with an emphasis on potential sources of confusion that we have heard from our students. Those of you who feel this information is already well digested may only require a quick read of this section. However, as most seasoned practitioners know, review is always useful, and you might even pick up a morsel or two that help you treat your next patient more effectively. For every reader at all levels of experience, that is our sincere hope.

In Chinese, the word for pattern is *zheng*. A pattern is the total constellation of a patient's signs and symptoms as gathered by the four examinations, including tongue and pulse signs. A disease or *bing*, on the other hand, is made up of a smaller group of symptoms which are believed to define that disease in all persons with it. Such disease-defining signs and symptoms are a disease's pathognomonic signs and symptoms or those by which it is specifically known. Thus, while a disease usually has a narrow definition of specific signs and symptoms, a pattern is the entire holistic *gestalt* of the patient. This includes objective signs and subjective sensations beyond those which are strictly pathognomonic of the patient's disease. In general, a disease's pathognomonic signs and symptoms only account for a percentage of the patient's entire pattern as seen by Chinese medicine.

Everyone with a certain disease must display certain key signs and symptoms before they can be diagnosed with that disease. For instance, patients with measles must display a characteristic rash, whereas patients with chicken pox must display characteristic pustules. However, a person with a disease may also display a large number of other idiosyncratic signs and symptoms. In Chinese medicine, these additional variable signs and symptoms are indications of the patient's constitution, their relationship of righteous to evil qi, and their idiosyncratic response to the disease.

Most systems of medicine, including other styles of non-TCM Chinese medicine and modern Western medicine, primarily base their treatment on the diagnosis of diseases. As a matter of fact, our first acupuncture teacher taught a disease-based treatment system. Two patients with certain key, pathogno - monic signs and symptoms are diagnosed as suffering from the same disease, whether this be systemic lupus erythema- tous or rheumatoid arthritis, measles or chicken pox, divertic- ulitis or appendicitis. Based on this disease diagnosis, these two patients are then given the same treatment because they suffer from the same disease.

The problem with this approach is that it does not take into account the patient's constitution, the relationship of their righteous to evil qi, or their idiosyncratic response to the dis- ease. Thus two people with the same disease may be given the same medicine, with one getting better and flourishing, while the other may fail to get better and develops all sorts of side effects. In the latter case, this is because only the abstract con- cept of the disease was addressed and not the totality of the actual patient with that disease.

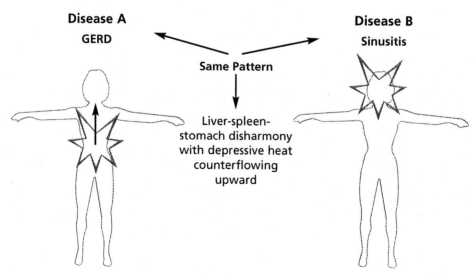

DIFFERENT DISEASE, SAME PATTERN

Disease A
GERD

Disease B
Sinusitis

Same Pattern

Liver-spleen-
stomach disharmony
with depressive heat
counterflowing
upward

Standard professional Chinese medicine also begins with a disease diagnosis. In contemporary professional Chinese medicine, that disease diagnosis may either be based on traditional Chinese disease categories, such as mounting, strangury, and welling abscess, or on modern Western disease categories, such as bronchial pneumonia, cerebroma, or lipoma.

However, the Chinese medical practitioner also makes a pattern discrimination and, in fact, emphasizes this pattern discrimination as the primary basis for treatment. Thus the famous dictum of Chinese medical methodology states:

Yi bing tong zhi
Tong bing yi zhi

Different diseases, same treatment
Same disease, different treatments

What this means in Chinese medicine is that two patients with the same disease will receive two different treatments *if their patterns are different.* While two patients with different

SAME DISEASE, DIFFERENT PATTERN, PART B

GERD	GERD
Patient 1	Patient 2

Esophageal reflux
Pattern A

Esophageal reflux
Pattern B

Large appetite
constipated, loud
voice, irritable

Poor appetite
loose stools, fatigued,
soft voice

**Male: works outside,
40 years old**

**Female: office worker,
55 years old**

diseases will receive the same treatment *if their patterns are the same.* This is the first fundamental thing to remember about the practice of professional Chinese medicine. Although it is important to make a disease diagnosis and to take the typical course of a disease and its peculiar characteristics into account, in standard professional Chinese medicine, it is more important to treat the pattern than the disease.

If one only sees the disease, it is like failing to see the forest for the trees. The disease is merely a figure within the ground of the total *gestalt* or pattern that is the patient. Therefore, the first step in writing a Chinese herbal prescription in standard professional Chinese medicine begins with a pattern discrimination. Almost without exception, when Western practitioners ask me what formula to use for their patient, they give me a disease diagnosis. Although that is the proper approach in modern Western medicine and its cousins, chiropractic and naturopathy, it is not the methodology of professional Chinese medicine. Thus, we must first discuss making a Chinese medical pattern discrimination as the primary necessary prerequisite for discussing how to write a Chinese herbal prescription.

> **In standard professional Chinese medicine, only arriving at a correct pattern discrimination rationally results in a correct treatment plan.**

The Four Examinations

Looking, Listening/Smelling, Questioning, Palpation

This information is organized in the following way:

Signs & Symptoms	Tongue Signs	Pulse Signs

Making a pattern discrimination

In standard professional Chinese medicine, only arriving at a correct pattern discrimination rationally results in a correct treatment plan. Since professional Chinese medicine bases its treatment primarily on the patient's personal pattern, it is imperative that this discrimination be as accurate as possible. At present, only information gained by the four (methods of) examination can be used to establish a Chinese medical pattern discrimination. These four are looking, listening/smelling, questioning, and palpation. However, when comparing patterns to each other, one mostly compares the A) signs and symptoms, B) tongue signs, and C) pulse signs. Thus the information gathered by the four examinations is typically organized into three groups of information.

It is the comparison of the total *gestalt* of signs and symptoms, tongue, and pulse which make up a pattern. These can be spoken of as the pathognomonic or ruling markers defining a pattern and differentiating it from all other patterns. For instance,

---

10 Types or Subsystems of Pattern Discrimination

1. Eight principle pattern discrimination (*ba gang bian zheng*)

2. Five phase pattern discrimination (*wu xing bian zheng*)

3. Viscera & bowel pattern discrimination (*zang fu bian zheng*)

4. Channel & network vessels pattern discrimination (*jing luo bian zheng*)

5. Qi & blood pattern discrimination (*qi xue bian zheng*)

6. Fluid & humor pattern discrimination (*jin ye bian zheng*)

7. Disease cause pattern discrimination (*bing yin bian zheng*)

8. Six aspect (or divisions) pattern discrimination (*liu fen bian zheng*)

9. Four aspect (or divisions) pattern discrimination (*si fen bian zheng*)

10. Three burner pattern discrimination (*san jiao bian zheng*)

---

in liver depression qi stagnation (*gan yu qi zhi*), the signs and symptoms may include chest oppression, frequent sighing, belching and burping, irritability, a darkish tongue with normal tongue fur, and a bowstring or wiry pulse. Whereas, in liver channel depressive heat (*gan jing yu re*), there may be many of these same signs and symptoms but there will also be differences. In this case, there will not only be belching but acid regurgitation. There will not just be irritability but even irascibility. The tongue will tend to be red with swollen edges and yellow fur, while the pulse will be bowstring and rapid. It is these different signs and symptoms that discriminate liver depression qi stagnation from liver channel depressive heat.

In standard professional Chinese medicine, there are 10 types or subsystems of pattern discrimination. Each of these subsystems has their own patterns with their own criteria and pathognomonic signs and symptoms. In clinical practice,

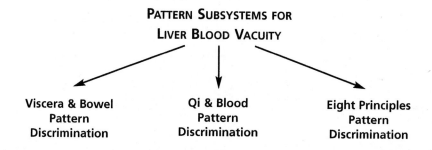

however, elements of patterns from one subsystem are typically combined with elements of another subsystem. For example, if a patient is discriminated as suffering from liver blood vacuity, this complex pattern is made up from elements of three of the above subsystems. Because the pattern is primarily associated with the liver, it is partially based on viscera and bowel pattern discrimination. Because it involves the blood, it is also partially based on qi and blood pattern discrimination. And because it involves vacuity, it likewise is partially based on eight principles pattern discrimination.

New practitioners are often confused as to which set of patterns to use in their discrimination of a particular patient. In Chinese medicine, one uses whatever combination of pattern discrimination matches the entirety of the patient's signs and symptoms most closely. In other words, one uses whichever one(s) fit the patient at hand. None of these subsystems of pattern discrimination is any better than any other. Each are like tools hanging on a workbench. If a certain job calls for a hammer, one uses a hammer. If another job calls for a screwdriver, one uses a screwdriver. Neither a hammer nor a screwdriver is intrinsically better than the other. However, one may work better for the job at hand. It is the same with Chinese medical subsystems of pattern discrimination. One should use whatever system most accurately describes their patient without any value judgements about the intrinsic merits of each.

For instance, many patients at the onset of the common cold are best described by warm disease theory, in which case a wind heat contraction with fever and sore throat may be seen as the defensive aspect or division of the four aspects pattern discrimination subsystem. However, the same patient who was first diagnosed according to warm disease theory may also be diagnosed several days later according to six divisions pattern discrimination if they exhibit alternating fever and chills with loss of appetite and fatigue. Later, that same patient may be discriminated as suffering from lung yin vacuity as their disease runs its course. This diagnostic label is a mixture of viscera and bowel and eight principles pattern discrimination. Yet this is in no way an inconsistency in the use of these systems. Each subsystem is merely made up of patterns of signs and symptoms and the goal is to find one or more patterns which accurately describes one's patient at that moment in time.

Thus these patterns are only pragmatic tools to help in providing discriminating treatment to individual patients. If one goes to a department store and tries on several brands of clothes, one may find that a size six in one brand is the same as a size seven in another. Within a single brand, a size six may be right and a size seven be wrong, but that in no way invalidates that in a different brand (or system) a size seven might be right.

The benefits of this methodology

Because this methodology treats each individual as an individual and also treats the entire *gestalt* of that person's being, its treatments are both safe and effective. Side effects are the result of not taking into account the idiosyncracies of an individual patient when prescribing. Although a certain medicine should, in theory, treat a certain disease in all people, because of individual differences in constitution as well as righteous and evil qi, some patients may tolerate that medicine and some people may become further imbalanced by it. If we know the Chinese medical description of a medicinal and the patient's pattern discrimination, then we should have a good idea of whether that medicinal will cause side effects or not, what those side effects will be, and whether or not those side effects are acceptable given the duration of that medicinal's expected length of administration.

> **If we know the Chinese medical description of a medicinal and the patient's pattern discrimination, then we should have a good idea of whether that medicinal will cause side effects or not, what those side effects will be, and whether or not those side effects are acceptable given the duration of that medicinal's expected length of administration.**

This system, when done well, should produce few if any side effects. Practitioners of Chinese medicine do not believe that, when it comes to medical treatment, it is alright to rob Peter to pay Paul. In Chinese medicine, the entire organism is seen as an interdependent whole. Side effects are a sign that a medicinal has caused an imbalance in a tissue, organ, or function.

Such side effects contradict Chinese medicine's holistic view of the body as a totally integrated organism.

In addition and as said above, a medicinal that works in one patient may not work in another. If I know the Chinese medical description of a given medicinal, I can also know in who it will work and why it works when it does. This is because a given medicinal must work within a real-life, individual human being and must work in coordination with the patient's own metabolism. The predisposition of the patient's metabolism is described by the Chinese medical pattern discrimination. Hence this methodology of basing treatment on each patient's personal pattern discrimination is not only safer but tends to be more effective than a purely disease-based prescriptive methodology.

Further, this methodology allows a practitioner to rationally explain to the patient why they got ill and the impact of their diet and lifestyle on the course of their illness. Patterns in Chinese medicine are based not only on empirical observation the way homeopathic patterns are. They are also based on theoretical concepts regarding disease causes and disease mechanisms. The name of every Chinese medical pattern implies a disease mechanism. For instance, if a patient is diagnosed as suffering from an external contraction of wind heat, the practitioner can counsel the patient to avoid drafts and getting chilled, avoid eating hot, spicy food, and avoid taking acrid, warm medicinals. Thus the patient is enlightened as to the cause of their disease and what they can do about its course. This empowers the patient and helps them participate in and take responsibility for their treatment.

Problems we encounter when doing a pattern discrimination

In our experience, Western practitioners commonly encounter several problems with this system of pattern discrimination. Certainly I encountered these problems myself as a young practitioner. First, because most of us must learn this system in translation, it's easy for us to miss the associations and cues which exist in Chinese.

What do I mean by this? A single Chinese word often has more than one meaning or connotation, each meaning having potential clinical implications that are difficult to capture when translated into a single English term. For instance, if I see the term *ni tai* translated as a "smooth tongue fur," which it is in some texts, I will not necessarily understand that this tongue coating is associated with an accumulation of dampness because the word "smooth" in English has no such connotation. Whereas, if this word is translated as "slimy tongue fur," which it also is in some texts, and I know how the tongue fur is created according to Chinese medical theory, this immediately should make logical connections with dampness and turbidity. Similarly, if I see the words *ru mai* translated as a "soft pulse," I may not understand this pulse's relationship to the accumulation of dampness. In this case, the alternate translation of "soggy" or "sodden" pulse makes that association with the relevant disease causes and disease mechanisms easier to understand. In Chinese, all these various associations are inherent within the words.

Secondly, no one Chinese medical textbook, whether in Chinese or English, is categorically complete when it comes to signs and symptoms associated with patterns. Each author tends to give a selection which they think most important or to simply write down what comes to mind first. Therefore, different authors give slightly different lists of representative signs and symptoms for the same patterns. If a Western student or practitioner has access to only a single textbook, they frequently are not aware of the wider range of signs and symptoms possibly associated with a given pattern.

And third, many English language translations of Chinese medical books fail to translate either fully or accurately the sections on disease causes and disease mechanisms. This information is what allows a practitioner to have an in-depth understanding of how each sign and symptom in their patient got there and, as such, is vital to our clinical thought process. Incomplete or faulty translation of this information may be due to a variety of reasons. As discussed above, since a single Chinese word may have several meanings, more than one of which has clinical significance, it can be difficult to render the often technical and abstruse language into what the translator perceives as meaningful English. Faced with this dilemma, the translator must choose one word which seems most suitable to them in the context at hand, leaving the other possible meanings out of the translation altogether. Further, some Western-oriented Chinese translators have told us they are concerned that the traditional Chinese concepts will look silly to Western medical professionals and so leave out sections they think will be unacceptable, write what they think a Western professional will find believable, or gloss them only briefly.

> **If one understands the disease mechanisms at work within a given pattern, one can posit, in the light of Chinese medical theory, what impact these mechanisms will have on the tongue, pulse, and various functions and tissues of the body.**

Why are disease causes and mechanisms so important to us? Because, if one understands the disease mechanisms at work within a given pattern, one can posit, in the light of Chinese medical theory, what impact these mechanisms will have on the tongue, pulse, and various functions and tissues of the body. In this case, we are not dependent upon lists of symptoms appearing in textbooks which are never totally comprehensive or categorically complete. Rather, we can account for particular signs and symptoms in our individual patient based on Chinese medical disease cause-disease mechanism theory. It is an understanding of disease causes and mechanisms that allows us to think flexibly and intelligently within the Chinese paradigm of patterns.

However, in order to do this, a practitioner must constantly keep in mind like their own name, address, and phone number all the fundamental statements of fact of Chinese medicine. For example, if I know without hesitation that the breast is circulated primarily by the stomach and liver channels, I can further logically deduce that distention and pain of the breasts may be a possible symptom of liver depression qi stagnation, even if my main textbook does not happen to mention this. Further, in order to be perfectly clear about this, I must know that the liver is in charge of coursing and discharging and that, when the liver is replete, it often invades the stomach via the control cycle of five phase theory. In addition, when I remember that the liver stores the blood, that the *chong mai* is the sea of blood, that the *chong mai* is one of the two most important vessels controlling menstruation, and that the *chong mai* connects with the stomach channel at *Qi Chong* (St 30), then I can account for the fact that breast distention and pain typically occurs prior to menstruation even though only specifically gynecological texts mention this symptom under liver depression qi stagnation.

In other words, in professional Chinese medicine, all the various facts we were asked to learn by heart in our introductory classes on Chinese medical theory become the sentences we use to describe what is going on in our patients. These facts become the propositions in the logical syllogism we create to prove to ourselves that we have arrived at the right conclusions about each patient. As a young practitioner, I did not think this level of memorization was vital. However, it was also my experience that when I went back and actually committed these statements of fact to the deepest part of my heart and mind, that was when I truly began to be able to practice this medicine with confidence and reliable success.

Statements of Fact Explaining Premenstrual Breast Distention and Pain Due to Liver Depression Qi Stagnation

Statement #1. The breast is circulated by stomach (foot *yang ming*) and liver (foot *jue yin*) channels.

Statement #2. The liver is in charge of the coursing and discharge of qi.

Statement #3. When the liver is depressed and its qi stagnant, it cannot do its function of coursing and discharging. It may become replete and hot.

Statement #4. When the liver is replete, it may invade the stomach.

Statement #5. The liver stores the blood.

Statement #6. The *chong mai* is the sea of blood.

Statement #7. The *chong mai* and *ren mai* control menstruation.

Statement #8. The *chong mai* connects to the stomach channel at *Qi Chong* (St 30).

Statement #9. If the liver is depressed and its qi is stagnant, qi may then become stagnant in the breast via the liver channel and the stomach channel, and the blood in the *chong mai* may become static. Since the *chong* and *ren* rule menstruation, these symptoms are likely to become worse during the build up of qi and blood in the lower burner prior to menstruation.

That being said, the other single most important thing that we can say about making a Chinese medical pattern discrimination is that no sign or symptom should be omitted simply because it does not seem to fit one's preconceived ideas about the patient's disease diagnosis. In the process of making a pattern discrimination, signs and symptoms gathered first often suggest a particular pattern to the practitioner. However, as we gather more signs and symptoms, some of these may not fit with our preconceived ideas about that pattern. In this case, we must think more deeply about the pattern discrimination and the disease mechanisms that could cause it until we come up with a pattern discrimination whose mechanisms do account for all the patient's signs and symptoms, perplexing and seemingly contrary or not.

> It was my experience that when I went back and actually committed these statements of fact to the deepest part of my heart and mind, that was when I truly began to be able to practice this medicine with confidence and reliable success.

Patients may, of course, require more than one pattern to describe their situation. While Chinese medical textbooks make it seem like patients exhibit very simple, discrete patterns, these single, neat diagnostic boxes or categories are merely teaching devices designed to highlight the differences between patterns. In real-life clinical practice, patients do not tend to manifest a single, textbook perfect, discrete pattern but rather a combination of elements of two, three, or even more patterns. In fact, based on my more than 20 years experience, I [BF] would say that most Western patients with the chronic diseases that tend to be our bread and butter in the world of alternative care display not less than three patterns and often as many as seven or eight simultaneously!

Reframing your patients' experience

In trying to unravel such a tangled skein of signs and symptoms, it is once again very important to first record the patient's signs and symptoms as completely and accurately as possible. This means sharpening one's abilities to see, hear, smell, question, and feel. In particular, one must ask questions which are designed to reframe the patient's experience into the terminology of Chinese medicine. For instance, if the patient is asked how their bowel movements are, they may say they are constipated. This can mean different things to different people. It is imperative that the practitioner clarify exactly what the patient means by this. Does it mean they do not have a bowel movement every day? Do they mean that defecating is difficult or uncomfortable? Or does it mean that the stools are hard and bound? Each of these different descriptions may potentially mean something different in terms of Chinese medical disease mechanisms and pattern discrimination.

Or a patient may say that they are depressed. This does not necessarily mean the same thing in Chinese medicine as it does in everyday English. Does the patient mean that they feel chest oppression, irritability, and frustration, or does it mean that they feel listless, fatigued, and cannot get out of bed? The difference between these two sets of symptoms is the difference between a correct and incorrect pattern discrimination. It is true that Chinese tend to somaticize their complaints and Western patients tend to psychologize theirs. Therefore, Western practitioners attempting to do Chinese medicine with Western patients must constantly keep in mind and also point out to their patients that all emotional experiences are simultaneously physically felt experiences. As Westerners, we tend to conceptualize and describe our feelings with abstractions: "I feel happy," "I feel sad," "I feel anxious," etc. Yet each of these abstract concepts are accompanied by (or are names we give to) physical feelings and sensations. We will have an easier time with pattern discrimination if we train ourselves and our patients to reconnect with these physical feelings in order to match up their complaints with Chinese, somaticized, pattern-differentiating signs and symptoms.

Mastery of pulse diagnosis

There is no shortcut to honing one's Chinese medical ability to gather accurate information via the four examinations. It simply takes time to sharpen these abilities. In particular, it may take years to really learn to read the pulse. Learning the pulse means developing the ability to consciously and consistently discriminate all of the 28 pulses. In my experience, simply knowing nine or 10 pulses—fast and slow, floating and sunken, bowstring, fine, or slippery—is not enough to do an accurate Chinese medical pattern discrimination on a complicated patient. In our typical patient population in the West, it is useful if not vital to be able to identify the surging, moderate/retarded, scattered, sodden/soggy, choppy, drumskin, scattered, short, and vacuous pulses at the least. In order to learn these, my experience says that we simply have to memorize their Chinese medical definitions verbatim and keep these in mind when feeling the pulse.

Let's again take the soggy pulse as our example. The definition of the *ru mai* or sodden/soggy pulse is that it is floating, fine, and soft or pliable. If I write down on the chart that the patient's pulse is floating, fine, and soft *but do not recognize this as the verbatim definition* of the soggy pulse, I will not necessarily associate this with the disease mechanisms associated with the soggy pulse. Although this ability is, in my experience, largely a function of time and maturation which cannot be rushed, it cannot even begin until the word for word definitions of the pulse images are committed to memory. When we have done this small amount of memorization, we have a better chance of being able to accurately describe what we feel under our fingers and to connect it with clinically meaningful disease mechanisms. In the welter of all we must remember to graduate from school, these definitions are easily forgotten once the exam for that class is passed. The good news is that this information is still available and we can go back and learn it again, as if we were re-loading the operating system on our computer to make sure it is working at optimal capacity. Further, it's important to realize that modern Chinese medicine has tended to downplay the pulse and to oversimplify its teaching. For instance, Hua Tuo, in his *Zhong Zang Jing (Classic of the Central Viscera)*, says over and over again that the slippery pulse is a vacuity pulse. Likewise, Zhu Dan-xi, in his *Dan Xi Zhi Fa Xin Yao (The Heart & Essence of Dan Xi's Methods of Treatment)*, says that the bowstring pulse is also a vacuity pulse. This is contrary to modern Chinese textbooks, but a vital piece of information when trying to understand chronically ill, complicated Western patients who often exhibit slippery, bowstring, surging, or floating pulses, all of which can be associated with counterflow inversion and underlying vacuity. Thus, in studying the pulse, it is more than a little helpful to study premodern Chinese texts as well as the modern literature available on this subject.

The arithmetic of pattern discrimination

Although I have heard some Western teachers of Chinese medicine say that the practitioner should "go with their gut feeling or intuition" about their patients' patterns, my Chinese teachers have all stressed that unraveling complicated patterns is based on very clear logic. In fact, doing a Chinese medical pattern discrimination is something like a mathematical problem, in that it is an additive process. When we work on a math problem, we are not allowed to simply leave out one or two of the numbers

> . . . doing a Chinese medical pattern discrimination is something like a mathematical problem, in that it is an additive process. When we work on a math problem, we are not allowed to simply leave out one or two of the numbers because it might make the problem easier to solve!

because it might make the problem easier to solve! Similarly, as mentioned above, we must be able to account for every sign and symptom in our pattern discrimination, without leaving out the ones that do not fit our initial hypothesis or that we cannot initially understand. For example, if the patient's tongue is red, this invariably signifies heat, at least in the upper burner since the tongue is in the upper burner. If the tongue fur is dry and yellow, the yellow signifies heat affecting the stomach qi and the dryness signals injury to stomach fluids. If the tongue is also fat with teeth-marks on its edges, this suggests an accumulation of body fluids. Since the spleen is the primary viscus in charge of the transportation and transformation of body fluids, this fatness and fluting suggest spleen vacuity and dampness. Thus an analysis of the tongue signs alone suggest that the patient is suffering from an element of heat causing drying of the stomach with a concomitant accumulation of dampness. All this can be and needs to be corroborated and further clarified by the pulse and other general signs and symptoms.

For me, it also helps to remember that very few symptoms can be ascribed a single, universal meaning. All but a handful of signs and symptoms may be the result of more than a single disease mechanism. When analyzing and ascribing meaning to any sign or symptom, that sign or symptom must be seen in relationship to all other signs and symptoms. For instance, night sweats are commonly due to yin vacuity and vacuity heat forcing fluids out of the body during the night which is ruled by yin. However, night sweats may also be due to heart blood vacuity, spleen vacuity with accumulation of dampness, and half interior-half exterior invasion of external evil qi. Further, a person may have yin vacuity and vacuity heat that is due to persistent damp heat with concomitant heart blood and spleen qi vacuity and dampness. Which of these mechanisms are operative in a given patient is determined by the total constellation of their signs and symptoms. But unless we can determine with accuracy which patterns we are treating, our treatment of the patient will be

Hallelujah Symptoms

While typically no one sign or symptom always indicates a single pattern in Chinese medicine, there are exceptions to every rule. The following is a list of our "**Hallelujah Symptoms.**" These are the handful of signs and symptoms in Chinese medicine which do only indicate a single pattern. For instance:

Fatigue - spleen vacuity
Drowsiness after eating - spleen vacuity
Dizziness standing up - spleen vacuity
A fat, enlarged tongue - spleen vacuity
Easy bruising - spleen vacuity
A bitter taste in the mouth - liver-gallbladder heat
Irritability - liver depression
Rib-side pain - liver depression
Sores on the lips - stomach heat
Rapid hungering, large appetite - stomach heat
Abdominal distention - qi stagnation
Sighing - qi stagnation
Night blindness - blood vacuity

When we say that these signs and symptoms only indicate a single pattern, we are not talking about disease mechanisms, nor are we talking about the complicated evolutions of these simple patterns. For instance, while lip sores always indicate stomach heat, stomach heat may be complicated by lung heat and/or heat toxins. While irritability always indicates liver depression, such depression may be associated with depressive heat, phlegm, phlegm heat, blood stasis, blood vacuity, qi vacuity, or even external contraction of wind evils. And, although textbooks typically say a fat, enlarged tongue indicates the accumulation of water dampness, since the spleen is averse to and damaged by dampness, if there is dampness causing an enlarged tongue, there will be spleen vacuity. Similarly, although fatigue is, *ipso facto*, a symptom of spleen qi vacuity, this may be due to and may result in phlegm damp encumbrance.

inaccurate a certain percentage of the time. Intuition and gut feelings may or may not help us, but a thorough knowledge of patterns and disease mechanisms will give us the surety to diagnose and prescribe with reasonable precision for each suffering individual who sits before us asking for our care.

> **Intuition and gut feelings may or may not help us, but a thorough knowledge of patterns and disease mechanisms will give us the surety to diagnose and prescribe with reasonable precision for each suffering individual who sits before us asking for our care.**

This means that the mechanism associated with any sign or symptom must be corroborated by related signs and symptoms. In the case above, if the pulse is rapid and slippery instead of fine, if the tongue fur is yellow and glossy instead of scant and dry, and if there is urinary urgency with burning, turbid, yellow urine, these signs and symptoms all suggest something other than or in addition to yin vacuity.

We all want to be clinically successful and do the best job for our patients. With that in mind, we cannot stress enough the importance of first accurately gathering signs and symptoms, then analyzing them individually, and eventually synthesizing them to reveal their Chinese medical meaning. To use an example already given above, a bowstring or wiry pulse most commonly indicates liver depression qi stagnation, more commonly abbreviated to just liver qi. A bowstring pulse plus a rapid pulse equals heat plus stagnation. Just in that way, we first take apart all the individual signs and symptoms and then add the indications back up again to arrive at what is most commonly a complex, multifaceted pattern discrimination. However, the difficult part is that, at the same time, the meaning of each individual sign or symptom is dependent upon the total constellation of signs and symptoms seen in relationship to each other. So the parts of the puzzle that each patient presents must be teased apart and then analyzed both separately and together to find their clinical meaning.

Very commonly in the West, our patients suffer from complex, recalcitrant diseases. As practitioners of a foreign, alternative system of medicine, our patients typically come to us after having tried numerous other practitioners and systems of treatment. Thus the easy or self-limiting cases are often winnowed out before they make it to our doors. To make matters worse, previous treatment itself may have caused iatrogenic complications, making the case even more difficult to unravel. This is especially the case if the patient is still taking one or more Western, Ayurvedic, homeopathic, and/or naturopathic medicines from some other practitioner(s). [See Chapter 12 for more on this subject.] In this case, we may have a hard time knowing what is the patient's underlying condition and what is a manifestation of the medication. Thus, it is not uncommon to come across patients with hot above and cold below, a hot, dry stomach and vacuous or cold, damp spleen, damp heat in their large intestine and vacuity cold affecting their kidneys, or heat and dampness mutually binding with qi and blood stasis and stagnation at the same time there is kidney yang vacuity and cold below and yin vacuity and heat above. Such complex presentations are common in our clinics here in the West and yet they would present a challenge to even the best Chinese practitioner with many years of experience!

Upon graduation from five years of medical school, Chinese practitioners are assigned to a large clinic or hospital. There they are given only patients whose diseases are commensurate with their level of knowledge and experience. In addition, there are always senior practitioners to give advice and critique and correct the young practitioner's diagnosis and treatment. This allows practitioners in China to develop their skill and knowledge slowly and in a relatively supportive environment. Here in the West, Chinese medical education is still in a developmental stage. It is shorter than what is required in China and has a far

more limited clinical component. Upon graduation, the most
common practice scenario in the West is a private, single practitioner clinic, without mentoring or clinical support. If the first
patient who knocks on our door after setting out our shingle is
someone with cancer, MS, or AIDS, how can we be expected to
understand these cases? Such patients tend to have complicated,
multifaceted, seemingly contradictory patterns and, in a
Chinese clinic, would be sent to the senior practitioners with
decades of clinical experience and knowledge.

For the reasons listed above, Western practitioners often
require more knowledge and insight in treating patients than
their Chinese peers. And yet, our educational system as currently designed cannot always start us off with all the skill
and knowledge we need. One way to improve this situation is
to read as widely in the literature on our own as possible. On
the one hand, for the bravest souls this means studying medical Chinese, since the overwhelmingly bulk of the literature
exists only in Chinese and will, for a variety of reasons, never
be translated into English. On the other hand, I personally
have found the theories contained in Li Dong-yuan's *Pi Wei
Lun (Treatise on the Spleen & Stomach)* to be the single most
helpful book in clarifying the contradictory but interrelated
mechanisms so often at work in our American patients. This
book goes beyond where modern Chinese textbooks leave off
and, even in China, practitioners are renewing their interest
in this book as containing many of the answers necessary to
treating complicated cases involving allergic hyperimmunity,
autoimmunity, hypoimmunity, endocrine dyscrasia, and
chronic, polysystemic candidiasis and intestinal dysbiosis.

Using treatment principles to improve our results

In Chinese texts, it is said that the treatment principles or *zhi
ze* are the bridge between the pattern discrimination and the
treatment or formula. In Chinese books and journals, after
the pattern discrimination there always comes a statement of
treatment principles. These are theoretical statements about

what needs to be done in order to rectify the imbalance implied by the name of the pattern. As such, they help to lead us to the correct chapter in our formula textbook. Such treatment principles are couched in the technical language of Chinese medicine and only certain principles are agreed to be the correct principles for the treatment of particular patterns.

For instance, if a patient's pattern discrimination is liver depression qi stagnation, the requisite and usual treatment principles for remedying this imbalance are to **course the liver, rectify the qi, and resolve depression.** Whereas, if a patient is discriminated as suffering from external contraction of wind heat, the treatment principles are to **resolve the exterior, diffuse the lungs, and clear heat** using acrid, cool medicinals. In the latter case as in many others, different Chinese authors may give slightly varying principles for the same pattern. However, when one looks at these variations more closely, they are mostly just different ways of saying the same thing or differences in therapeutic emphasis. For instance, in the second example above, some authors might say that external contraction of wind heat requires one to **relieve or resolve the exterior, dispel wind, and clear heat.** Nonetheless, although there is some latitude in stating one's treatment principles, this latitude is circumscribed and we can say that certain treatment principles are either correct or categorically wrong for the treatment of certain patterns.

Chinese medical practitioners regularly use between 200-300 treatment principles. [See Appendix II for a list of the most commonly used treatment principles.] Typically, there will be one treatment principle for each element of the pattern diagnosis. For example, if a patient suffers from liver blood vacuity, one should **supplement the liver and nourish the blood.** Thus there is one principle for the liver and another for the blood. In this way, both elements implied by the pattern's name are comprehensively and categorically addressed. Chinese authors most commonly write these principles in four syllable groups. For instance, if a patient suffers from spleen-kidney yang vacuity, the treatment principles might be stated in Chinese, *jian pi yi qi, bu shen wen yang.* This means to **fortify the spleen and boost the qi, supplement the kidneys and warm the yang.**

As with so much of Chinese medical technical terminology, the words used in constructing treatment principles often have associations not readily apparent in translation. For instance, the word *zi* means to enrich and is only used in relationship to yin. Its character includes the water radical. One may come across the construction, *zi shen,* to enrich the kidneys. In Chinese, this implies enriching kidney yin or water (not kidney yang, kidney qi, or kidney essence). For an English-speaking practitioner to really understand the implications of these words, it helps to spend some time studying the terminology used in stating treatment principles and learning such technical associations which are apparent in Chinese.

Most of the time, therapeutic or treatment principles are addressed to the *ben* or root of the imbalance implied in the pattern's name. Sometimes, however, if *biao* or branch treatment of acute signs or symptoms must be given, this is also specified in the treatment principles. Since vomiting involves a loss of fluids, the finest essence of the digestate, and qi, vomiting is a branch symptom that, in Chinese medicine, is accorded priority or at least prominence in treatment. Therefore, if there is vomiting, one typically appends the words **stop vomiting** to the preceding list of treatment principles. Similarly, one appends the principles of **stop diarrhea** for diarrhea, **stop bleeding** for any type of hemorrhaging, **stop pain** for any kind of severe pain, etc. When such branch treatment principles are included in a list of treatment principles, this *requires* that the practitioner address this symptom specifically and symptomatically. This process will become clearer in the next chapter when we discuss modifications of formulas.

CHAPTER 2

Writing a Formula
That Works for Each Patient

In Chapter 1, we've reviewed the basics of analyzing your patients according to the process of Chinese medical diagnosis. In this Chapter, we move from diagnosis into the realm of treatment using Chinese herbal medicine. We continue from where we ended in Chapter 1, with the importance of treatment principles.

Getting to the right formula category

In the methodology of professional Chinese medicine in China, both the treatment principles and the pattern discrimination are a charting requirement. Why should this matter to us? It matters because the treatment principles help *funnel* us toward the correct formula and its proper modification. Using liver depression qi stagnation again as our example, if a patient suffers from liver qi, the usual therapeutic principles are to **course the liver and rectify the qi**. Once I have written those words down underneath the pattern discrimination, it then becomes crystal clear, accord-

> In the methodology of professional Chinese medicine in China, both the treatment principles and the pattern discrimination are a charting requirement.

ing to the logic and methodology of Chinese medicine, that I should chose a formula from the qi-rectifying category of formulas.

In Chinese medicine, there are 20 some different categories of formulas, such as exterior-resolving formulas, phlegm-transforming formulas, blood-quickening formulas, blood-stopping (*i.e.*, stop bleeding) formulas, etc. Chinese formulas and prescriptions texts are organized and group their formulas according to these categories. Thus the principle of **rectifying the qi** immediately directs me to the appropriate group of formulas from which to chose. This narrows down my choices from

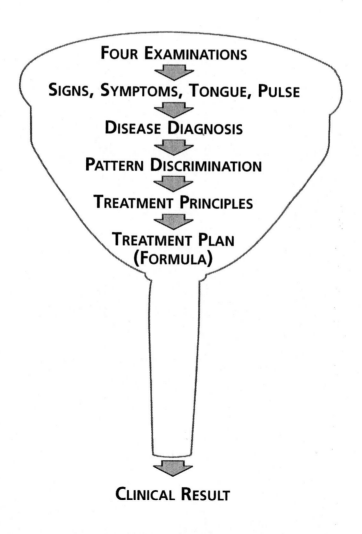

FOUR EXAMINATIONS

SIGNS, SYMPTOMS, TONGUE, PULSE

DISEASE DIAGNOSIS

PATTERN DISCRIMINATION

TREATMENT PRINCIPLES

TREATMENT PLAN
(FORMULA)

CLINICAL RESULT

potentially hundreds of formulas to a much smaller, more manageable group. This is especially so if I stick with a repertoire of the most standard, best known Chinese medical formulas.

Within the qi-rectifying category of formulas, I next look only at those formulas which **course the liver**, since that is the other principle stated for the treatment of liver qi. Out of the total of qi-rectifying formulas, this narrows down my choices even more. Now I have only a small handful of formulas from which to chose. If the pattern is truly this simple, I would next look for the formula which not only **rectifies the qi and courses the liver** but which is known through empirical experience to treat the disease or signs and symptoms of the patient before me. The standard formula for this very simple scenario is *Si Ni San* (Four Counterflows Powder).

Formula for these Treatment Principles: *Xiao Yao San*
Ingredients:
Chai Hu (Radix Bupleuri)
Bai Shao (Radix Albus Paeoniae Lactiflorae)
Dang Gui (Radix Angelicae Sinensis)
Bai Zhu (Rhizoma Atractylodis Macrocephalae)
Fu Ling (Sclerotium Poriae Cocos)
mix-fried *Gan Cao* (Radix Glycyrrhizae Uralensis)
Bo He (Herba Menthae Haplocalycis)
Sheng Jiang (uncooked Rhizoma Zingiberis Officinalis)

Chai Hu (Radix Bupleuri)
Zhi Shi (Fructus Immaturus Citri Aurantii)
Bai Shao (Radix Albus Paeoniae Lactiflorae)
Gan Cao (Radix Glycyrrhizae Uralensis)

However, such a simple pattern discrimination among Westerners is the exception rather than the rule. Since liver depression qi stagnation is a species of repletion, based on five phase theory, the viscus and bowel of the earth phase are most

Western disease diagnosis: Amenorrhea
Chinese disease diagnosis: Menstruation behind schedule
Symptoms: Fatigue, irritability, craves sugar, easy
nausea, scanty, infrequent menstruation
Pulse signs: Soggy (*i.e.*, floating, fine, forceless),
bowstring in the right *guan*
Tongue signs: Fat with teeth-marks, pale
Pattern dx: Liver depression qi stagnation,
spleen vacuity and dampness with
blood vacuity
Treatment principles: Course the liver
and rectify the qi, fortify the
spleen, eliminate dampness,
and nourish the
blood

vulnerable to disease transmission. Thus, if the liver qi has led
to spleen vacuity weakness complicated by blood vacuity and
an element of dampness, I must find a formula which **courses
the liver, rectifies the qi, fortifies the spleen, eliminates dampness, and nourishes the blood.** The most famous formula whose
ingredients categorically and comprehensively accomplish all
these goals is *Xiao Yao San* (Rambling Powder).

If there are all of the above elements in the patient's pattern
discrimination, but the patient's liver qi has become

depressed to the point of transforming into heat, then one must also add the principles: **clear heat and resolve depression**. In that case, one is directed to *Dan Zhi Xiao Yao San* (Moutan & Gardenia Rambling Powder) since it includes two ingredients to clear heat from the liver and the blood which the liver stores. In most formula and prescription texts, including Bensky and Barolet's *Chinese Herbal Medicine: Formulas & Strategies*, this formula appears as a modification of *Xiao Yao San* as the standard formula.

> *Dan Pi* (Cortex Radicis Moutan)
> *Zhi Zi* (Fructus Gardeniae Jasminoidis)
> *Chai Hu* (Radix Bupleuri)
> *Bai Shao* (Radix Albus Paeoniae Lactiflorae)
> *Dang Gui* (Radix Angelicae Sinensis)
> *Bai Zhu* (Rhizoma Atractylodis Macrocephalae)
> *Fu Ling* (Sclerotium Poriae Cocos)
> mix-fried *Gan Cao* (Radix Glycyrrhizae Uralensis)

On the other hand, if blood vacuity is more pronounced along with the liver qi, spleen vacuity, and dampness, then one is directed to *Hei Xiao Yao San* (Black Rambling Powder) since this version of this standard formula includes *Shu Di* (cooked Radix Rehmanniae Glutinosae) to more specifically and effectively aid *Dang Gui* and *Bai Shao* in nourishing the blood. This is also usually listed under *Xiao Yao San* as a modification of that formula.

> *Shu Di* (cooked Radix Rehmanniae Glutinosae)
> *Dang Gui* (Radix Angelicae Sinensis)
> *Bai Shao* (Radix Albus Paeoniae Lactiflorae)
> *Chai Hu* (Radix Bupleuri)
> *Bai Zhu* (Rhizoma Atractylodis Macrocephalae)
> *Fu Ling* (Sclerotium Poriae Cocos)
> mix-fried *Gan Cao* (Radix Glycyrrhizae Uralensis)
> *Bo He* (Herba Menthae Haplocalycis)
> *Sheng Jiang* (uncooked Rhizoma Zingiberis Officinalis)

To review this process, it was the statement of the principle to **rectify the qi** that leads to the qi-rectifying category of medicinals in this case. From there, the further principles stated lead one with ever greater precision and narrowing down of choices to the precise formula within that category. Most commonly, the key principle that leads us to the correct category of formulas is the first principle stated or, at least, is within the first pair. In the example above, **coursing the liver** usually precedes the principle of **rectifying the qi**. This is probably just because of the way these four syllables sound to the Chinese ear. Nonetheless, it should be remembered that each principle is usually made up of two Chinese words and two such principles comprising four syllables are read as a unit.

Therefore, in the case of external contraction of wind heat, **resolving the exterior** is the first and most important principle. This leads us to the exterior-resolving category of formulas. **Clearing heat** is subsidiary to that and further refines and narrows the search for an appropriate formula within that category.

Going back to the liver, if a patient displays signs and symptoms consistent with liver wood invading earth and a hot, replete stomach and vacuous, damp spleen, one might say that the treatment principles are to **course the liver and rectify the qi, fortify the spleen and eliminate dampness, and clear stomach heat**. However, loss of harmony between the liver and spleen and spleen and stomach can also be treated by the principle of harmonizing. In such a case, the treatment principles can also be to **harmonize the liver and spleen and spleen and stomach while clearing heat from the stomach and eliminating dampness**. If one states it this way, then those principles lead one to the harmonizing (*he ji*) category of formulas. Within that category, the standard and most famous formula which categorically and comprehensively embodies and addresses each of these principles is *Xiao Chai Hu Tang* (Minor Bupleurum Decoction).

Western disease diagnosis: GERD
Chinese disease diagnosis: Stomach pain
Symptoms: Heartburn and acid reflux, fatigue, irritability, craves sugar, rapid hungering, bad breath
Pulse signs: Fast, soggy (*i.e.*, floating, fine, forceless), bowstring in the right bar
Tongue signs: Fat with teeth-marks, red tongue body with dry, yellow fur
Pattern dx: Liver-spleen disharmony, spleen dampness with stomach heat
Treatment principles: Course the liver and rectify the qi, fortify the spleen, clear heat and eliminate dampness

Formula for these Tx Principles: *Xiao Chai Hu Tang*
Ingredients:
Chai Hu (Radix Bupleuri)
Ren Shen (Radix Panacis Ginseng)
Ban Xia (Rhizoma Pinelliae Ternatae)
Huang Qin (Radix Scutellariae Baicalensis)
mix-fried Gan Cao (Radix Glycyrrhizae Uralensis)
Da Zao (Fructus Zizyphi Jujubae)
Sheng Jiang (uncooked Rhizoma Zingiberis Officinalis)

We know that this formula does address and embody each of these therapeutic principles by recognizing and understanding the Chinese medical rationale for the inclusion of each ingredient in this formula. When we know the materia medica well enough to immediately comprehend what each ingredient is meant to do in the formula, we will have no trouble understanding exactly what pattern and, therefore, what patient a formula fits.

In this last example above, although the treatment principles do lead to the correct category within which to find the correct formula, our theoretical understanding of Chinese medicine does have to be good enough to know that liver-spleen and spleen-stomach imbalances are described as *bu he*, lack of harmony and that, therefore, it is necessary to pick a formula from the harmonizing category.

> **If our foundation in Chinese medical theory is sound and we have studied the formulas within each traditional category so that we have an overview of the contents of these categories, this system of selecting formulas is extremely logical, safe, and effective.**

Although there are some tricky aspects to finding formulas within the traditional categories of formulas based on therapeutic principles in turn based on pattern discrimination, if our foundation in Chinese medical theory is sound and we have studied the formulas within each traditional category so that we have an overview of the contents of these categories, this system of selecting formulas is extremely logical, safe, and effective. As stated above, when problems exist in making this system work, they are mostly due to not understanding this system as it is understood in Chinese where the correct associations are made by the language itself. Even studying a little medical Chinese can greatly help this situation. Such problems may also arise because of not being adequately familiar with the traditional categories of formulas and the most important formulas within each category.

Thus, if a patient's presenting pattern discrimination is blood stasis, we then write down under that the requisite treatment principles which are to **quicken the blood and transform stasis**. These principles imply, according to Chinese medical logic, that we should look for an appropriate formula under the blood-rectifying or *li xue* category of formulas. Within that category, we then select a formula which quickens the blood and transforms stasis in the appropriate part of the body. For instance, *Ge Xia Zhu Yu Tang* (Below the Diaphragm Stasis-dispelling Decoc- tion) primarily dispels blood stasis in the hypochondral regions. Whereas, *Shao Fu Zhu Yu Tang* (Lower Abdomen Stasis-dispelling Decoction) is especially effective for dispelling blood stasis in the lower abdomen.

Similarly, if the patient's pattern discrimination is phlegm accumulation, then the treatment principle is to **transform phlegm**. Hence we should look under the phlegm-transforming category of formulas. If the phlegm is hot phlegm, we look for a formula that **transforms phlegm *and* clears heat**. If the phlegm is cold phlegm, we look for a formula that **transforms phlegm *and* eliminates dampness**. Then, within those various categories of formulas, we must also look to see that the formula has been found to be empirically effective for the

---

CHART WRITING PROCESS REVIEW

Patient's Major Complaint
Disease Diagnosis (Both Western & Chinese)
Distinguishing Signs & Symptoms, Tongue, Pulse
Pattern Discrimination
Treatment Principles
Guiding Formula
Additions, Subtractions

particular patient's disease diagnosis, addresses their signs and symptoms, and especially addresses their major complaint. Once we take all these factors into account, it is hard not to arrive at a formula which fits the patient's disease, pattern, and signs and symptoms.

Writing a good Chinese medicinal formula

Although the process of moving from a pattern discrimination to a statement of treatment principles greatly helps in identifying the correct category of formulas in which to search, when we have found a standard guiding formula, we will still usually have to modify it in order to tailor it as perfectly as possible to the patient's needs. In China the practitioner first writes down on the patient's chart their major complaint or already established disease diagnosis. Then comes the main distinguishing signs and symptoms including the tongue and pulse using the standard, professional, technical vocabulary of Chinese medicine. These are followed by the pattern discrimination and the treatment principles. Then the practitioner writes the name of the formula. Most of the time in clinical practice, the name of the formula is modified by either of two pairs of words. Either the words *jia wei*, added flavors, or the words *jia jian*, additions and subtractions, are prefixed or suffixed to the formula's name.

Added flavors mean added ingredients. Additions and subtractions mean that some ingredients of the standard formula have been deleted and others which are not part of the standard formula have been added. Sometimes Westerners are under the mistaken impression that, since most of the medicinal ingredients used in Chinese internal medicine are herbs, this system is safe for that reason. However, many of these ingredients are very potent and others are used in comparatively high doses. What makes this system safe and effective is the precision in writing and modifying formulas to fit patients as exactly as possible. If an ingredient in a standard formula is not necessary, it is just as important to take this out since it may very well cause side effects or iatrogenesis. If Chinese herbs are powerfully good in the right situation, then it is axiomatic that they can also be powerfully bad in the wrong situation. Thus, it is just as important to delete unnecessary ingredients as to add additional ingredients when modifying a formula.

> **What makes this system safe and effective is the precision in writing and modifying formulas to fit patients as exactly as possible.**

Liu Wei Di Huang Wan (Six Flavor Rehmannia Pills) is one of the best known formulas in modern Chinese medicine. It is designed for the treatment of kidney yin vacuity. Of its six ingredients, three are supplementing to the kidneys and three are draining. Two of the draining ingredients seep and eliminate dampness. The third draining ingredient clears vacuity heat and heat in the blood. The ingredients of this formula are:

> *Shu Di* (cooked Radix Rehmanniae Glutinosae)
> *Shan Zhu Yu* (Fructus Corni Officinalis)
> *Shan Yao* (Radix Dioscoreae Oppositae)
> *Fu Ling* (Sclerotium Poriae Cocos)
> *Ze Xie* (Rhizoma Alismatis Orientalis)
> *Dan Pi* (Cortex Radicis Moutan)

Of these ingredients, the first three are the three kidney-supplementing ingredients, and the last three are the three draining ingredients.

Because the kidneys are one of the three viscera which govern water metabolism and, in particular, control urination, patients with kidney yin vacuity frequently have urinary disturbances. With kidney yin vacuity, we commonly expect short, frequent, yellow urination, terminal dribbling, and/or nocturia. However, not all patients suffering from kidney yin vacuity do suffer from urinary complaints. The Chinese medical idea of the kidneys covers a number of other tissues and functions besides urination. If a patient is diagnosed as being kidney yin vacuous but they do not have any irregularity in their urination, the two water-seeping, dampness-eliminating medicinals are deleted in contemporary Chinese practice. Because *Ze Xie* and *Fu Ling* seep water, they can drain righteous qi and yang. Therefore, not only can they cause fluid dryness if used unnecessarily, but they can also result in qi vacuity.

In this formula, *Dan Pi* is meant to clear heat which may arise from supplementing kidney yin. Since kidney yin and yang are mutually interdependent, if yin is supplemented, yang may also flare up and, in particular, enter the blood aspect or division. In addition, this ingredient also quickens the blood. It is included in this formula because blood stasis is a common complicating factor in the types of chronic diseases associated with kidney yin vacuity. However, quickening the blood may unnecessarily damage the blood, while clearing heat unnecessarily may damage the spleen and stomach, the postnatal root of qi and blood production, or diminish the righteous warmth of the lifegate fire, the source of all transformation in the body.

In Chinese clinics, we may still write on a patient's chart that the guiding formula employed was *Liu Wei Di Huang Wan* if only the three supplementing ingredients are used. Then, in addition, there may be another 12 ingredients added. In this case, the formula is written, *Liu Wei Di Huang Wan Jia Jian* (Six Flavors Rehmannia Pills with Additions & Subtractions). A new herbal practitioner looking at such a formula may find it hard to recognize the resulting formula as *Liu Wei Di Huang Wan* at all.

Ingredients are added to standard formulas in order to A) augment and amplify certain functions of the formula, B) treat disease mechanisms (*i.e.*, complicating patterns) not covered by the standard formula, and C) to treat specific symptoms.

For instance, *Huang Qi* (Radix Astragali Membranacei) and *Dang Shen* (Radix Codonopsitis Pilosulae) may be added to *Xiao Yao San* discussed above in order to further supplement the spleen and boost the qi. *Che Qian Zi* (Semen Plantaginis) might be added to this formula in order to augment the elimination of dampness through seeping water or promoting urination. We have seen how *Shu Di* can be added to further nourish and enrich the blood. Whereas, *Huang Qin* (Radix Scutellariae Baicalensis) may be added to *Dan Zhi Xiao Yao San* to clear heat from the lungs and *Mai Men Dong* (Tuber Ophiopogonis Japonici) might be added to moisten lung dryness if prolonged depressive heat floating upward has accumulated in the lungs damaging lung fluids. In this case, these two ingredients are added to treat complications of the main disease mechanisms to which this formula's standard ingredients are targeted. Or, we may add *Ju Hua* (Flos Chrysanthemi Morifolii) and *Bai Zhi* (Radix Angelicae Dahuricae) to treat the symptoms of headache located in the eyes and across the brows of the forehead due to depressive heat flaring upward. But we might add *Chuan Xiong* (Radix Ligustici Wallichii) to treat the symptoms of a temporal headache, especially on the right side.

In particular, if we add any of a number of treatment principles beginning with the word *zhi* or "stop" to the list of stated principles, we must add ingredients specifically to address those acute branch symptoms. As mentioned above, these include vomiting, sweating, diarrhea, bleeding, loss of essence such as from spermatorrhea or abnormal vaginal discharge, and relatively severe pain. All these are seen as very debilitating and harmful to the long-term health of the patient. They need to be stopped as quickly as possible. Therefore, ingredients are added to the formula which are known to have a powerful, pronounced effect on the particular symptom. For instance, excessive bleeding during menstruation may be due to depressive heat entering the blood aspect. There it causes the blood to move frenetically outside its pathways and causes it to overflow beyond measure. In this case, we may use *Dan Zhi Xiao Yao San* as the guiding formula. But, based on the treatment principles of stopping bleeding, we should also add blood-stopping medicinals, such as *Di Yu* (Radix Sanguisorbae Officinalis) and *Qiang Cao Gen* (Radix Rubiae Cordifoliae). Both of these medicinals not only stop bleeding but they do so by specifically cooling the blood according to Chinese medical theory.

Organizing our formulas

If we begin with a standard formula as a basis or guide, we do not have to worry too much about such traditional organizing principles as ruler, minister, envoy, and assistant. Nevertheless, it is useful to recognize which ingredients play such roles within any formula. This can help in choosing a formula to begin with and in making modifications after a formula is picked. The sovereign ingredient is the main ingredient intended to accomplish the main treatment principle. In writing a prescription, this ingredient should be listed first. According to Li Dong-yuan, this ingredient should also be used in the largest amounts, although in contemporary Chinese medicine this is not always the case. The ministerial ingredients are those which aid and extend the functions of the ruling ingredient, while the assistants usually are meant to accomplish allied functions or address specific symptoms. Envoy ingredients are those which carry or target the effects of the rest of the ingredients to a specific viscus, bowel, channel, tissue, or body part.

For example, in the famous formula, *Bu Zhong Yi Qi Tang* (Supplement the Center & Boost the Qi Decoction), *Huang Qi* (Radix Astragali Membranacei) and *Ren Shen* (Radix Panacis Ginseng) are the sovereigns. They supplement the qi and fortify the spleen. Mix-fried *Gan Cao* (Radix Glycyrrhizae Uralensis) and *Bai Zhu* (Rhizoma Atractylodis Macrocephalae) are the ministers. They also supplement the qi and fortify the spleen. *Dang Gui* (Radix Angelicae Sinensis) nourishes the

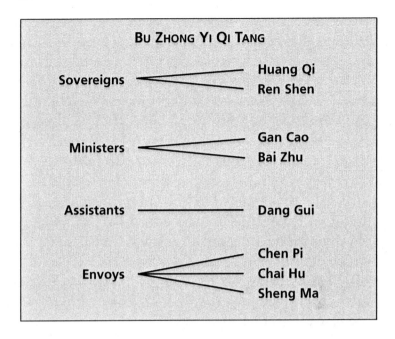

BU ZHONG YI QI TANG

Sovereigns —— Huang Qi / Ren Shen

Ministers —— Gan Cao / Bai Zhu

Assistants —— Dang Gui

Envoys —— Chen Pi / Chai Hu / Sheng Ma

blood. Since the blood is the mother of the qi, the addition of *Dang Gui* helps support the engenderment of qi. This ingredient, therefore, assists the previous four indirectly. And *Chen Pi* (Pericarpium Citri Reticulatae), *Sheng Ma* (Rhizoma Cimicifugae), and *Chai Hu* (Radix Bupleuri) are the envoys. *Chen Pi* descends turbidity, while *Chai Hu* and *Sheng Ma* upbear and lift clear yang.

If necessary, one can also add assisting ingredients to address complicating disease mechanisms and their symptoms. For instance, for prolapse of the rectum or uterus, one can add *Zhi Shi* (Fructus Immaturus Citri Aurantii) to the above. Or, in order to treat urinary frequency and incontinence, one can add *Che Qian Zi* (Semen Plantaginis) and *Ze Xie* (Rhizoma Alismatis) if due to spleen dysfunction and *Shan Yao* (Radix Dioscoreae Oppositae) and *Wu Wei Zi* (Fructus Schizandrae Chinensis) if due to complicating kidney vacuity.

Determining the right dosage

Although most Chinese medical textbooks and formula compendia give standard or suggested dosages for each formula, the issue of dose is one which requires discussion. If we look at the dosages listed for a standard Chinese formula such as *Liu Wei Di Huang Wan* discussed above in a modern Chinese medical book such as Him-che Yeung's *Handbook of Chinese Herbs and Formulas, Vol. II* and then compare these to the Japanese *kanpo yaku* dosages of the same formula listed in Hong-yen Hsu's *Commonly Used Chinese Herb Formulas with Illustrations*, we will see that the standard professional Chinese dosages are roughly three times more across the board than the *kanpo yaku* dosages. This same discrepancy is apparent if we look at the dosages of standard formulas as listed in the premodern sources in which they first appeared and their modern Chinese doses compared in Bensky & Barolet's *Chinese Herbal Medicine: Formulas & Strategies*. In general, modern Chinese medical doses are three or more times higher today than in premodern times.

This discrepancy between *kanpo yaku* doses and modern Chinese doses can be explained by the fact that *kanpo yaku* practitioners prescribe set formulas with little modification. Since the formulas they use, the so-called *jing fang* or classical prescriptions, come from the Han dynasty and are revered as divine revelations, Japanese practitioners tend to regard them as sacrosanct set pieces. If one formula does not work, another entire formula is chosen. In addition, *kanpo yaku* practitioners emphasize treating the root or *ben* as opposed to addressing the branches of a disease. They seem to prescribe relatively simple formulas in small doses to be taken over a protracted period of time with slow, steady improvement on the part of the patient.

Modern professional Chinese practitioners, on the other hand, see their patients each week. They do not regard the formulas they use as sacrosanct and inviolable. And they try to achieve relatively speedy relief of all the patient's branch symptoms at the same time as addressing their disease mechanism's root cause. Thus, modern Chinese medical practition-

ers tend to prescribe highly modified and fairly complex formulas at much higher doses per individual ingredient.
The discrepancy between the smaller ancient Chinese doses
and larger, modern Chinese doses for the same formulas are
more difficult to explain. Is it possible that contemporary
patients are sicker than their premodern peers and thus
require routinely larger doses? Or is it possible that due to
leaching of the soil and overcultivation, Chinese medicinals
are not as potent as before. This is not a question we feel we
can answer.

Typically in the People's Republic of China today, most ingredients in most formulas are dosed at either nine or 10 grams.
These numbers are derived from the old, premetric system of
weights and measures. In that old system, three *qian* was a
standard dose for ruling and ministerial ingredients, two *qian*
for assistant ingredients, and one *qian* for envoy ingredients.
One *qian* is slightly more than three grams. Therefore, some
practitioners routinely prescribe nine grams for the main
ingredients in their formulas and others prescribe 10 grams.
Those that stick to nine grams do so, in part, because nine is
an odd or yang number just as three *qian* is. Those Chinese
practitioners that prefer to use 10 grams tend to also be those
most influenced by modern Western medicine. Personally, I
prescribe mostly on the basis of multiples of 3 – 1.5, 3, 4.5, 6,
9, 12, 15, 18, 21, etc. However, this should be recognized for
what it is, a somewhat arbitrary convention based on theory
and numerology, not on chemistry.

In a modern Chinese medicinal formula, when more than 9-
10 grams of an ingredient are prescribed, there are usually
either of two factors at work. First, if a branch symptom is
severe, a larger than normal amount of an ingredient may be
used. Thus, if qi vacuity is severe, one may use 12, 30, or even
60 grams of *Huang Qi* (Radix Astragali Membranacei). In this
case, *Huang Qi* may or may not be the ruling ingredient.
Secondly, some ingredients are simply known to be effective

at higher than the usual doses. For instance, *Pu Gong Ying* (Herba Taraxaci Mongolici Cum Radice) and *Bai Jiang Cao* (Herba Patriniae Heterophyllae) are routinely prescribed at 21-30 or more grams per packet because those are the doses at which they become effective. Typically, these ingredients are not the ruling ingredients in the formulas in which they appear.

Likewise, when less than 9-10 grams of a single ingredient are prescribed in a modern Chinese medicinal formula, this is usually due to similar reasons. Either the ingredient is merely adjunctive, functioning as an envoy or assistant, or it is so strong-acting and even potentially toxic that it has been determined that only a certain smaller dosage is necessary and advisable. In addition, standard dosages of certain ingredients may be reduced if it is understood that, in a given patient, based on their pattern discrimination, that ingredient is likely to cause unwanted side effects or iatrogenesis.

Therefore, although there are standard dosages used in modern Chinese medicine for most ingredients in most formulas, the exact amounts of any ingredient in any formula are a matter of judgement on the part of the prescribing practitioner. That is why, in many Chinese medical books, dosages are not given for any ingredients in any listed formulas. In deciding on the dosage of each and every ingredient in a formula, the practitio-ner is expected to know and understand why the ingredient is in the formula and, further, how much of that ingredient in the formula our individual patient needs and can tolerate. In other words, we must have a firm grasp of the materia medica with all the medicinals' flavors, temperatures, channel

> **Although there are standard dosages used in modern Chinese medicine for most ingredients in most formulas, the exact amounts of any ingredient in any formula are a matter of judgement on the part of the prescribing practitioner.**

gatherings, functions, indications, combinations, contraindications, and usual dosage ranges. We need to become so acquainted and conversant with the Chinese medicinals that we can immediately know why any ingredient is in any formula. Then it is relatively easy to decide how much of that ingredient a specific patient should be given.

Some Western practitioners feel that the contemporary Chinese norm of 9-10 grams per ingredient per packet is arbitrary. Some feel it is too much or unnecessary. However, in reviewing the modern Chinese medical journal literature, it seems to me that the dosages of individual ingredients prescribed in China are tending to be even higher than 9-10 grams per ingredient. It is not uncommon today to see the majority of ingredients in a formula listed at 12-15 grams per ingredient per day. In my experience, however, most Western patients simply cannot afford the cost of such large *bao* or packets. Typically, I use nine grams per ingredient as my standard dose per packet which I have the patient spread out over a two day period. For the majority of my patients this compromise allows them to get results, if perhaps slower than otherwise, at a price per day they can afford. I frequently would like to give higher doses but only do so in extraordinary situations or for serious branch symptoms and short durations.

At some point, I do think we as practitioners should do comparative studies measuring the effectiveness of different dosages on a single patient population. Until that time, deciding on exact dosages per ingredient must depend on personal knowledge and experience and on an assessment of what the consumer can afford.

Other factors that can and should be taken into account when deciding upon dosages are the season, weather, and prevailing geographic environment and the patient's age, sex, size, and constitution. Li Dong-yuan, in his *Pi Wei Lun (Treatise on the Spleen & Stomach)*, gives much interesting advice on the modification and adjustment of dosages of formulas based on the season and weather. For instance, some herbal practitioners suggest that the dosages of *Si Wu Tang* (Four Materials Decoction) be altered for each of the four seasons. This standard formula consists of:

> *Dang Gui* (Radix Angelicae Sinensis)
> *Bai Shao* (Radix Albus Paeoniae Lactiflorae)
> *Shu Di* (cooked Radix Rehmanniae Glutinosae)
> *Chuan Xiong* (Radix Ligustici Wallichii)

In the spring, yang qi rises upward and it is important that the liver's control of coursing and discharge be freely and easily flowing. Therefore, one might consider doubling the dosage of *Chuan Xiong* during the spring. During the summer, the weather is hot and one may sweat profusely. Patients requiring this formula have a tendency to be blood and yin vacuous and insufficient. Therefore, one might consider doubling the amount of *Bai Shao* in the summer. This medicinal is cold and also astringing, thus tempering the heat of the season and controlling perspiration. Fall is the season of dryness, and blood and body fluids share a common source. Therefore, one might consider doubling the amount of *Dang Gui* in this formula in the fall. And finally, the winter is the season of the kidneys and a time of storing essence. *Shu Di* not only nourishes the blood but supplements the kidneys and fulfills essence. Thus one might consider doubling *Shu Di* in the winter. The rationale behind these seasonal modifications is based on understanding the nature and uses of each ingredient and the tendencies and requirements of each season when seen from the perspective of the typical patient needing *Si Wu Tang*.

Obviously, infants and children should be given reduced dosages. This may be calculated by body weight. We can, in general, prescribe the same percentages of adult doses of each ingredient as the proportion of the child's weight to an adult's. We can also administer Chinese herbal decoctions to infants and small children by the dropper. Most American children will not drink even a quarter cup of an herbal decoction if given in a cup. However, they will drink the same decoction if squirted into their mouth via a dropper. In this case, we can give smaller but more frequent doses through the day rather than 2-3 larger doses.

Decocting & administering bulk-dispensed Chinese medicinals

Chinese society was, until the last 50 years, by and large, a sedentary, agrarian society. Patients of Chinese doctors lived nearby. They cooked their meals three times per day. Therefore, they came to depend upon decoctions or *tang* (literally soups) as their major method of medicinal administration. This is in contradistinction to nomadic Tibetans and Mongols who primarily came to rely on pills and powders.

There are a number of different methods of making a Chinese decoction. In fact, every teacher with whom I have studied Chinese medicine has had their own, slightly different method. The method I use with my patients is to simmer the herbs in six cups of water till they are reduced to approximately three cups. If there are shells or minerals in the decoction, these should be decocted for 30-45 minutes in advance before the other ingredients are added. If there are various aromatic substances in the formula, these may have to be added at the end of the cooking for the last 5-7 minutes. These include *Sheng Jiang* (uncooked Rhizoma Zingiberis Officinalis), *Gou Teng* (Ramulus Uncariae Cum Uncis), *Chuan Xiong* (Radix Ligustici Wallichii), *Mu Xiang* (Radix Aukandiae Lappae), *Yan Hu Suo* (Rhizoma Corydalis Yanhusuo), and *Sha Ren* (Fructus Amomi) to name a few of the most common such ingredients. Some flowers, such as *Hong Hua* (Flos Carthami Tinctorii) and *Ju Hua* (Flos Chrysanthemi Morifolii) should only be steeped at the end. The various gelatins, such as *E Jiao* (Gelatinum Corii Asini) and *Lu Jiao Jiao* (Gelatinum Cornu Cervi), should be broken up first and then dissolved in the hot liquid after the liquid has been strained and the dregs removed. Certain resinous powders, on the other hand, such as *Hu Po* (Succinum), should be chased down when drinking the decoction. In addition, some very small ingredients need to be placed in cotton muslin bags during decoction so that they do not get caught in or irritate the throat when drinking the decoction. This includes *Pu Huang* (Pollen Typhae), for instance.

Using the method above, one makes up six half-cup doses every two days and stores these for use in a clean, lidded, glass jar. If the weather is not too hot, this can be stored without refrigeration for the 36-48 hours necessary till it is used up. If the decoction is meant to clear heat, it may be drunk at room temperature. If the decoction is meant to supplement yang or warm the interior, it is best if each dose is reheated. Some American practitioners allow their patients to make up even 4-5 days' decoction at a time. However, my experience is that the flavor of stored decoctions changes after 36-48 hours. This change in flavor suggests to me that the decoction itself has undergone a chemical change and is no longer the same physical substance. Therefore, I have no assurance that it will have the same, intended effect. Because of this, I recommend my patients to only make up two days' supply of decocted herbs per time.

If I want my patients to get a higher, more potent dosage of decocted herbs, another method I sometimes use is to cook one *bao* or packet as above but with only three cups of water. This results in 1 1/2 C of decoction, or a one day's dose at 1/2 C, three times per day. However, instead of discarding the dregs, I tell the patient to reserve them in the refrigerator. The second day, the patient makes up a new bag of herbs just like the day before. Again they reserve the dregs. On the third day, they take the dregs, combine them, and recook them the same way to get a third day's dose from the ingredients of the two combined packets.

A somewhat similar method of stretching a single *bao* or packet of medicinals is to decoct it twice and then pour together the resulting two decoctions. However, in the People's Republic of China, most patients use only one *bao* per day. The method I was taught in Shanghai was to place the medicinals in a teapot and cover the medicinals with cold water one inch or so above the top of the medicinals. These medicinals are then allowed to soak for one hour. Then they are decocted for 45 minutes. After decoction, they are decant-

INGREDIENT	COOKING METHOD	SAMPLE INGREDIENTS
SHELLS & MINERALS	Simmer for 30-45 minutes prior to adding main ingredients	*Mu Li* and *Long Gu*
GINSENGS	Simmer whole roots separately for 30-45 minutes. Then eat the ginseng root. Add liquid to main ingredient liquid.	*Ren Shen*
MOST MEDICINALS	Simmer in 6 cups down to 3 cups for 30-45 minutes	
AROMATIC MEDICINALS	Add during the last 5-7 minutes of cooking	*Sheng Jiang, Gou Teng, Chuan Xiong, Mu Xiang, Yan Hu Suo, Sha Ren*
FLOWERS	Steep after the heat is turned off for 5 minutes	*Hong Hua* and *Ju Hua*
GELATINS	Dissolve in the hot liquid	*E Jiao* and *Lu Jiao Jiao*
RESINOUS POWDERS	Put in mouth and chase down with decoction	*Hu Po*
FINE POWDERS	Place in a muslin bag when cooking so that powders are not difficult to drink	*Pu Huang*

ed and the liquid reserved to be drunk in three measured doses within a single day. When I asked about reserving the dregs and recooking them, I was told that the peasants would rather throw the dregs on the road, thus symbolically casting the disease out of the house, there to be crushed by the wheels of passing buses and trucks.

It is important to remember and to explain to patients that making their Chinese herbal decoctions is no more time-consuming or difficult than cooking a pot of rice. In fact, I recommend that patients cook their decoctions when they are cooking dinner. If the patient says that they never cook their dinner from scratch but either always eat out or eat ready-to-serve, microwavable food, that in itself is a major problem with which the practitioner is going to have to deal. In my opinion, it is hard to be really healthy if we do not eat primarily a diet of freshly purchased, freshly cooked food. If a patient takes the time, as they or at least someone in their family should, to prepare at least one meal per day from scratch, then it is little extra trouble to cook their Chinese medicinals at the same time.

Time of administration

Traditionally, decoctions whose actions are primarily directed at the upper burner are taken after a meal. Because the stomach is full, the medicinals' actions are blocked from entering the lower burner. Thus decoctions for the treatment of cough or headache might be taken after meals. Conversely, decoctions whose actions are directed at the lower burner are taken on an empty stomach directly before a meal. When the meal is eaten, this "pushes down" the medicinals to the lower burner. Medicinals meant to supplement the kidneys are commonly specified to be taken before meals. However, in the People's Republic of China today, these guidelines are often dismissed as feudal superstition. At the clinics in China in which I worked, patients were routinely told to take their decoctions 15-30 minutes before meals.

However, sometimes the medicinals themselves can be too harsh for the stomach and cause nausea or cramping. In that case, the patient should be instructed to take the decoction after meals on a full stomach. If that alleviates the discomfort, then the patient should continue taking the decoction in that method. If that does not alleviate the stomach upset, the formula should be discontinued or modified so that it does not damage the stomach.

When decoctions are meant for the treatment of insomnia, it is best to take them later in the day so that the last dose is taken not long before going to bed. That may mean that the first dose is not taken till noon. Sometimes also, we may come across precise instructions in the literature about the preparation and administration of a certain formula. For instance, an author may state that the formula is to be taken in two even doses per day rather than three. Generally, I follow such instructions unless I am very familiar with the formula in question and know from experience that it is alright to administer on a different schedule.

If I tell a patient to take their decoction three times per day before meals, the question will inevitably arise about what to do if they skip a meal or eat only twice per day. In that case, I recommend that they simply take their third dose at a time evenly spaced from the others. Directions for taking their medicine either before or after meals only suggest when they should take their medicine in relationship to their meals. It does not mean that they should only take their medicine twice per day if they only eat two times that day. It is also possible to take 1 1/2 cups in two evenly divided doses rather than in three if one has forgotten to eat, does not plan on eating, or has forgotten to take their previous dose. Patients should be reminded that their medicine does no good sitting in a jar on their counter but only after they drink it. Rather than being too tightly wrapped about a dosage and administration schedule, it is better to simply take the medicine one way or another.

Duration of administration

At the Yue Yang Hospital in Shanghai where I did my clinical internship in the practice of Chinese internal medicine, patients were routinely sent home with seven days' supply of medicinals even after the first visit. Because the dispensing of the packet of medicinals is a labor intensive activity and once the medicinals are put in a packet or bag they cannot easily be separated back out, it is difficult to accept returns of formulas that have not worked as expected. However, it is important to remember that one's initial diagnosis is only a working hypothesis. It is only after the patient has taken their formula based on this hypothesis that we may confirm or modify that diagnosis. Therefore, I routinely only prescribe 2-4 days' dose after the initial visit. After that time, the patient checks back in with me and I ask if there have been any side effects. If there are any side effects, I then either further modify the formula or reconsider my diagnosis and guiding formula altogether.

If the formula is well selected and crafted for the individual, its bad taste should be abating by the third or fourth day. There should be no side effects, and the patient should begin to experience some ameliorating effect. If that is the case, then I prescribe the same formula for another 6-8 days. Because I usually prescribe one *bao* for two days, the majority of my patients check back in with me and renew their prescriptions every eight days instead of seven as in China. For acute cases, patients may only have to take a formula for one, two, or three days. For chronic cases, they may have to take decoctions for several months. When treatment must span a relatively long period of time, the practitioner should, in general, use medium to small doses, take care not to damage the spleen and stomach, and also give the patient regular breaks from taking decoctions altogether. Since I mainly treat women for gynecological complaints, commonly my patients without pronounced menstrual pain or excessive bleeding do not take herbs during their periods.

Once a chronic problem has been brought mostly under control, the practitioner may chose to switch their patient to a pill or powder. In this case, consistency over a long period of time is

Once a chronic problem has been brought mostly under control, the practitioner may chose to switch their patient to a pill or powder.

more important than making many modifications or administering large, fast-acting doses. Pills and powders are easy to take and help to secure the therapeutic results achieved by the stronger, faster acting decoctions.

Except for unusual circumstances, I never prescribe a single version of a decoction for more than eight days at a time. This is because people and the world are always changing. The seasons are changing, the weather is changing, the moon is changing, a person's mood, social life, sexual activity, and work are always changing. People have crises, change jobs, lose lovers and friends, take vacations, move to a new house, and catch cold, and it is important that their decocted medic-inals reflect and take into account all those changes. Unlike modern Western medicine which is so disease-oriented, Chinese internal medicine is treating not only the patient's disease but their entire pattern, and a Chinese medicinal decoction does not distinguish between the patient's root and branch since the medicinals enter the system as a whole.

Therefore, for me it is important not to prescribe a single for-mula for too many days. The formula should be written to be commenced the day the patient checks in with their practi-tioner. It is written based on their entire *gestalt* on that day as presented by their signs and symptoms, tongue, and pulse. If the patient waits to take the medicinals for several days, who knows what changes will intervene in the meantime? It is also important to explain to patients that if they are being treated for a chronic complaint and they experience an acute flare-up of some other problem, such as the flu or gastroenteritis, they should discontinue their medicine during that acute episode. At that time, the formula for their chronic complaint is not correct for their entire pattern, and, as stated above, if one's internal Chinese herbal medicine is not right based on their pattern discrimination, it is likely to cause side effects and iatrogenesis. In that case, it is best if the patient comes in and has a new diagnosis and a new prescription written for them during their acute episode. If that is not possible, they should at least be instructed to discontinue their medicinals until their symptoms have gone back to being the same as when the formula for their chronic problem was written.

Because Western patients are used to taking one medicine for one disease no matter what else is going on with them, Western practitioners of Chinese medicine need to be very clear about this with our patients. Our patients need to be informed that their decoction is treating them in their entirety and is not simply addressing their major complaint. This, in fact, is the beauty and power of professional Chinese medicine. I personally recommend writing a paragraph about this issue on whatever written handout the practitioner provides their patient instructing them how to make and take their decoctions. (See Appendix 4 for an example of an herbal instruction form.)

Conclusion

I have found individually prescribed Chinese herbal medicine dispensed from bulk and administered in decoction to be ex - tremely effective medicine. Contrary to the opinions of many Western practitioners, I have not found the majority or even a significant minority of my patients resistant to this form of medication. The ability to tailor the ingredients of a formula to the exact needs of a patient and the potency of bulk-dispensed, freshly decocted medicinals are such important and effective parts of using Chinese herbal medicine that I hope Western students and practitioners will seriously consider this methodology. Although desiccated extracts and ready-made pills have their place in the practice of Chinese internal medicine, the prescription and administration of so-called raw herbs has always been and, in my opinion, should continue to be the professional standard of care in Chinese medicine, whether in China or the West.

If the practitioner does not have any hesitation about prescribing decoctions, it is my experience that neither will patients be hesitant to drink them. If, on the other hand, the practitioner is apologetic about prescribing decoctions and suggests that there is an easier, more comfortable way to take their medicine, of course patients will pick up and act on their practitioner's ambivalence. For me [BF], the benefits of decocted medicinals far outweigh whatever their inconvenience, and I do not present my patients with an option. More importantly, I myself take Chinese herbal decoctions on a regular basis and mind neither their taste nor the making of them. Consequently, I have not found it difficult to have a thriving practice with hundreds of middle class American patients taking their Chinese herbs without complaint or problems with compliance.

> **If the practitioner does not have any hesitation about prescribing decoctions, neither will patients be hesitant to drink them.**

Problem Based Learning Exercises (See App. IV for answers)

1. What questions might a practitioner ask to corroborate a pattern discrimination of stomach heat with spleen qi vacuity dampness? What pulse signs might you expect to find?

2. What signs and symptoms would a practitioner look for to determine the specific pattern of night sweats presenting in their patient?

   A. yin vacuity and vacuity heat forcing fluids out of the body during the night

B. heart blood vacuity plus spleen vacuity with accumulation of dampness

C. half interior-half exterior invasion of external evil qi

D. yin vacuity and vacuity heat that is due to persistent damp heat with concomitant heart blood and spleen qi vacuity and dampness

3. If a patient's pulse is bowstring and slow, what pattern(s) does that suggest and what questions would you ask to determine the pattern? What other signs and symptoms would you look for? What disease mechanisms may account for a slow pulse?

4. For a patient with:

- a hot, dry stomach
- a vacuous, cold, damp spleen
- damp heat in their large intestine
- vacuity cold affecting the kidneys

What questions would you ask and signs or symptoms would you look for to corroborate each of these patterns?

What would you expect the pulse to feel like? If the spleen vacuity and dampness is at the heart of these patterns, what formula might you start with and how would you modify it?

5. What other symptoms might you look for in patients with kidney yin vacuity?

6. What medicinals could be added if the patient manifested intense low back pain and night sweats?

7. If a patient has a soggy pulse and slimy tongue fur, what other signs and symptoms would you need to find to corroborate a pattern of spleen qi vacuity weakness causing it to be unable to transform and transport body fluids?

Case History Exercises

Case 1: Female, 37 years old

The patient complained of mid-cycle bleeding for four months. At the time of this bleeding, the blood was scanty in amount and bright red in color. It was not accompanied by abdominal pain or any other symptoms except night sweats. Her menses were otherwise regular at 27-28 days with scanty, bright red blood lasting only three days. The woman was of slim build with small secondary sexual characteristics and prematurely grey hair. She also reported that menarche had not occurred till she was 16 and a half and that she had bouts of recurrent amenorrhea until she was 22. Her facial complexion was somewhat flushed red, and she seemed agitated or restless, stirring constantly. The patient's tongue was red with scanty fur, and her pulse was fine and rapid. Other signs and symptoms included a tendency to low back pain, frequent, darkish, but scanty urination and nocturia at least once per night. There was no pain or burning with urination. The patient's menstrual periods were unaccompanied by pain, and she did not have any PMS to speak of. If anything, she felt more restless and generally hot at the end of and directly after her period. The patient did say that she drank a good bit of coffee, smoked cigarettes, and also smoked marijuana pretty regularly.

1. What are the three causes of any and all pathological gynecological bleeding?
2. What happens in terms of *Chinese* medicine gynecology at mid-cycle?
3. What is/are this woman's pattern(s)?
4. What signs and symptoms indicate what pattern(s)?
5. What do the slim frame and underdeveloped secondary sexual characteristics indicate?
6. What role do the smoking of cigarettes, marijuana and drinking coffee, play in this case?
7. What should the treatment principles be for this case?
8. When should treatment commence and how long should it last each cycle?
9. Please write a representative formula for this case.

Case 2: Male, 57 years old

The patient complained of urinary difficulty at night. He would get up 2-3 times each night with a need to urinate. However, his stream was difficult to begin, was thin and forceless, and ended without completely evacuating the bladder. The man said that during the day, his urination was pretty normal, although sometimes he had terminal dribbling and a feeling of incomplete emptying. However, there was no pain or burning with urination, nor was it cloudy or turbid and his urine was a normal, light yellow color. The man was of mesomorphic build and looked reasonably healthy for his age. Other signs and symptoms included chronic low back pain made worse by overwork and fatigue, some generalized fatigue and loss of strength, somewhat decreased libido, perhaps a little difficulty hearing as well as he used to, a fat tongue with teeth-marks on its edges, and a fine, deep pulse in both cubit positions.

1. What are the two main causes of any and all inhibition of urination?
2. What is the significance of this man's urination being more difficult at night?
3. What is the man's probable Western disease diagnosis?
4. What should you advise this man to do in order to be a responsible professional caregiver?
5. What is/are the pattern(s) presented by this patient?
6. What role may the saying, "Enduring disease enters the network vessels," play in this case?
7. What are the treatment principles appropriate for this case?
8. What form of Chinese medicinals should this man be prescribed and why?
9. Please write a representative formula for this case.

Case 3: Female, 42 years old

The patient said that she had recently been diagnosed with interstitial cystitis via cystoscopy. The clinical symptoms that had prompted this diagnosis were frequent urination, a mild discomfort and pressure in her lower abdomen, and occasional urinary urgency. When asked to describe the feeling in her lower abdomen, the woman said that it was a heavy, sagging or downward pulling feeling. All these symptoms tended to be worse when the patient was fatigued. In addition, the patient's symptoms were worse before and during menstruation, and she sometimes had dyspareunia. Other signs and symptoms included premenstrual breast distention and irritability, premenstrual fatigue, a craving for sweets, a tendency to loose stools, and a tendency to hemorrhoids whenever she stood for a long time. The patient's menses tended to be heavy, and she reported orthostatic hypotension. Her tongue was fat with teeth-marks on its edges and thin, white fur, and her pulse was fine and bowstring.

1. What is this woman's Chinese medical disease diagnosis?
2. What is/are this woman's presenting pattern(s)?
3. Which signs and symptoms indicate which pattern(s)?
4. What does the orthostatic hypotension and recurrent hemorrhoids signify?
5. What is dyspareunia and what does it signify?
6. What is the key statement about any and all pain in Chinese medicine?
7. What are the treatment principles for this case?
8. What form of Chinese medicinals should this woman be administered and why?
9. Please write a representative formula for this patient.

Case 4: Female, 25 years old

The patient said that she had had premenstrual acne for the last several years. This acne was worse before her menstruation. It also occurred when the patient ate too much greasy, fried, and fatty foods. Because of her age, she also tended to drink a fair amount of alcohol. This young woman's menstruation tended to be late at 35-40 days, was medium in quantity, dark in color, and somewhat thick in consistency. Other premenstrual symptoms included irritability, breast distention and pain, lower abdominal bloating, and constipation with dry, hard stools. The patient was at day 26 in her cycle and had acne currently. The acne was mainly located around her mouth and along her chin. The pimples were red in color and some had developed pustules. There was no purple discoloring and there was no scarring or subdermal nodulations.

When questioned, the patient said that she had a tendency to bleeding gums as well as to bad breath. Her tongue was a dark, dusky color with dryish, yellow fur. Her pulse was bowstring and rapid and surging in the inch positions.

1. What is the first thing in making a pattern discrimination for a dermatological condition?
2. What channel were this patient's pimples primarily located on?
3. Given a physical description of the pimples themselves and their location, what is your disease mechanism hypothesis?
4. What signs and symptoms confirm this hypothesis?
5. Do any signs or symptoms deny this hypothesis?
6. What is/are this woman's presenting pattern(s)?
7. What are the treatment principles based on the foregoing pattern(s)?
8. Please write a representative formula for this case.
9. Do you think any dietary recommendations need to be made in this case? If so, what are they and why?

Case 5: Female, 45 years old

The patient had a recurring red, swollen, painful right knee joint for the last several months. She had been checked by a rheumatologist for autoimmune disease but the outcome was negative. The knee tended to swell and become more painful and red before this woman's menstruation each month which occurred every 27-30 days. It was also worse with damp, hot weather and if she ate fatty, greasy, fried and/or spicy, hot foods, which she often did. There was also a seeming relationship to sugar intake. Besides the gonarthralgia, the patient said she was constantly fatigued, was irritable before her menstruation, and tended to have loose stools also before and with menstruation. When questioned about these loose stools, she said that they were a light mustard color, were odorous, and left a burning sensation around her anus. This woman also revealed that she had a chronic, cheesy vaginal discharge with occasional vulvar itching and pain. If she ate a lot of hot, spicy food and drank alcohol, she could have burning urination for a couple/few days. There was a fat, reddish tongue with teeth-marks on its edges and yellow, slimy fur on its root. The patient's pulse was slippery, bowstring, and rapid overall, but was more bowstring and slippery in the cubit positions.

1. What type of impediment pain was this patient manifesting?

2. What other patterns was she also presenting?

3. How do you know that? Which signs and symptoms indicated what?

4. What are the treatment principles for this patient's disease plus pattern(s)?

5. Please write a representative formula for this patient.

6. Do you have any dietary recommendations for this patient?

7. How do you explain the disease mechanisms at work in this case?

Case 6: Male, 1 year-old

The patient was a little boy with recurrent earaches, and he was currently having an earache at the time of his examination. The child cried frequently from the pain, tugged and batted at his ear, and his face got red when he cried. The child had a fever known by both his skin and body temperature. The baby's pediatrician wanted to put the child on antibiotics. The child had been on several different antibiotics in the past for this problem. They worked temporarily, but then the earaches soon came back. If this continued much longer, the MD had said they would have to consider putting in tubes. The little boy was plump, had a blue vein at *Shan Gen* (the root of the mountain between his eyebrows), and a dark, reddish, and engorged index finger vein in the windgate position. The patient's mother reported that the child had always been colicky as an infant and that the earaches had begun when the child had first teethed. The mother had subscribed to the La Leche League's theory of feeding on demand. The child had recently lost interest in breast-milk except for his before bedtime feeding. The child loved sugar and sweets, and his mother gave him a lot of fruit juice believing it was "full of vitamins." Other favorite foods were refined flour cookies and crackers and ice cream. The child tended to be on the constipated side with dark, smelly stools. The mother also said the child often had bad breath.

1. What does a blue vein at *Shan Gen* indicate on an infant?
2. What does a dark, reddish, engorged vein indicate in the wind gate on the index finger of an infant?
3. What does bad breath indicate in an infant?
4. What is/are the presenting pattern(s) in this child?
5. What are the appropriate treatment principles for this case?
6. What tip or branch condition(s) require(s) its/their own treatment principle(s) in this case?
7. Please write a representative formula for this child. Be sure to take into account any principle formulated for any branch or tip conditions.
8. How are you going to have the mother administer this formula?

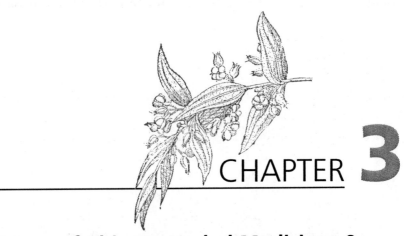

CHAPTER **3**

Forms of Chinese Herbal Medicines & Their Appropriate Use

Chinese herbal medicines come in a number of different forms, and there are standard conventions in professional Chinese medicine about these various forms and their different usages. There are two main divisions of Chinese herbal medicines. These are individually written, bulk-dispensed, water-based decoctions and ready-made medicines. Ready-made medicines intended for internal administration are then further divided into pills, tablets, capsules, powders, and tinctures.

Water-based decoctions
Water-based decoctions made from individually written, bulk-dispensed Chinese medicinals are the professional standard of care in the remedial treatment of disease in the People's Republic of China. The two main advantages of such water-based decoctions are 1) individually tailored prescriptions to fit the patient's exact needs and 2) relatively high dosages for speedy results. When I say high dosages, the average standard daily dose per medicinal in such a decoction is 9-10 grams. Since such decoctions commonly have 10-18 ingredients, total daily dosages run from 100-200 grams or more. It is not at all unusual to have prescriptions for decoctions made from 300 grams of herbs per day.

Even though it may be the standard of care in the People's Republic of China there are drawbacks to using water-based decoctions. These include: 1) high price depending on the country and the clinic, 2) labor intensive preparation in the dispensary, 3) cooking and preparation at home by the patient, 4) smell during the cooking process, 5) frequently unpalatable taste, and 6) patient compliance. In some countries where the price of bulk Chinese herbs is comparatively low, water-based decoctions are actually the cheapest way to get high therapeutic doses of Chinese medicinals. However, in countries where bulk Chinese herbs are not as readily and cheaply available (due either to Value Added Tax (VAT) or small market size), such water-based decoctions can be prohibitively expensive. In addition, the mark-up of the dispensary can also make a great difference in the affordability of this option. When looking for options to decrease this cost such as suggesting the patient use a single packet for two days or use two packets for three days, you should be aware that this does reduce the dosage available to the patient and does somewhat defeat the purpose of using water-based decoctions. In some cases, such a reduction in dosage or potency will not be an issue. In other cases, such as in acute conditions or diseases accompanied by severe conditions, such a reduction in potency may be unacceptable.

In China, patients being treated with bulk-dispensed, water-based decoctions are not typically treated with acupuncture at the same time. Because of the typical combination of these two therapies in the West, practitioners may find that they do not need to prescribe the high doses considered standard in the PRC. Nevertheless, in complex, multi-pattern conditions, it is difficult to match the prescription to the individual patient's needs unless we write an individualized formula, and water-based decoctions allow exactly this ability. Although there is not much that can be done about the smell of the Chinese herbs while cooking, it is a common experience for patients to report that a prescription which initially tasted terrible has come to taste OK after some time and that they even have come to crave their regular doses. This suggests that the body somehow recognizes the beneficial effects of the prescription. Typically, the cooking of a Chinese medicinal decoction takes from 20 minutes to one hour, and, during this time, the patient can be doing other things. There are automatic Chinese herb cookers available that make this process somewhat easier, and dispensaries can purchase (for around $3,000.00 U.S.) bulk Chinese herb decoctors that individually package each dose in plastic pouches. This is an interesting option for busy clinics. It allows patients to go home with precooked decoctions that can be stored in the refrigerator for use and then opened and drunk one at a time.

Ready-made Chinese medicines

As stated above, there are a number of different forms of ready-made Chinese herbal medicines. Traditionally, such ready-made medicines were primarily used for any of four main purposes: 1) over-the-counter self-medication, 2) long-term use in chronic, slowly changing conditions, 3) prevention, or 4) in the case of emergencies where one did not have the time to wait for the preparation of a water-based decoction. Even in China, compliance with water-based decoctions is an issue over extended periods of time. Therefore, when the practitioner knows the patient is going to have to take a prescription for a long time, they often may turn to one or another form of ready-made medicine. It is also common for Asian laypersons to first try an over-the-counter (OTC) remedy on their own before seeing a professional practitioner. If the OTC remedy works, great. If it does not, then they come to the clinic. Ready-made remedies are also prescribed by professional Chinese medical practitioners in order to prevent a relapse after a condition has been successfully treated with water-based decoctions. This is referred to in the Chinese medical literature as "securing and consolidating the therapeutic effects." For instance, after all the symptoms have disappeared due to the administration of decoctions, it is common for a Chinese practitioner to switch to a pill form of some version of the same formula for another couple of weeks to several months.

Pills

In Chinese medicine, most ready-made pills are made from either ground, powdered herbs bound together with water, honey, or some other medium or low-potency extracts. The advantage of pills are that they are easy to store, keep for a relatively long time, and are easy to dose and take. Their drawbacks are their low potency and their inability to modify other than by combining with yet other pills. Such a low potency may not be an issue when patients are being treated concomitantly with acupuncture-moxibustion and/or tuina. However, in many cases, such a low potency is a problem, meaning that the patient is unable to notice any beneficial results even after weeks or months of taking the pills.

In general, I would advise each practitioner to consider raising the dosages stated on the packaging of ready-made Chinese herbal pills, whether those pills are made in Asia, the U.S., or elsewhere. Manufacturers tend to state the low end of the dosage range to avoid overdoses by well-meaning laypersons and the potential legal suits that such overdosages may cause. Especially if we are attempting to remedially treat an active disease, we should consider raising the printed dosages. In doing this, we should take into account the patient's age and weight, whether the condition is acute or chronic, and the severity of the symptoms. In clinical practice, this may mean doubling, tripling, or even quintupling the stated dosages. At some point, this usually becomes cost-prohibitive and the patient balks at taking so many pills.

Tablets & capsules

Chinese herbal tablets and capsules tend to be made from higher potency extracts. These extracts are typically made from a dual water and alcohol extraction process with or without fillers and binders. The benefits of tablets and capsules are the same as those of pills, but their higher potency does help deliver more medicine. And, in the capsule form the medicine is bio-available much more rapidly. Their main drawback is also similar to pills. You cannot modify their ingredients. In addition, tablets and capsules usually have a shorter shelflife and are easily destroyed by exposure to excessive moisture. The dosages stated on the packages of Chinese herbal tablets and capsules also tend to be low. Therefore, practitioners must decide on the dosage for any given patient individually using the same criteria as stated above. But, it is possible with higher potency tablets and capsules to approximate the dosage of high-potency decoctions without an excessive number of tablets and capsules. Such tablets and capsules are often a good compromise therapeutically between high-potency decoctions and low-potency pills.

Powders

There are two main types of powders: 1) ground bulk herbs and 2) powdered extracts. Ground bulk herbs simply mean powdered bulk herbs. Such simple powders were traditionally used in Asia for either of two purposes. One, formulas could be made and stored for emergency use. At the time of use, the powder is then steeped in boiling water for 3-7 minutes and the resulting "tea" drunk, or they could be swallowed directly and chased with water. Secondly, powdered formulas could also be made for long-term use. In this case, the patient steeps a certain amount of the powder in boiling water each time they need to take a dose and drinks the resulting tea. This eliminates the time and effort of making a decoction. Thus it increases compliance in some patients. The drawbacks of ground bulk herbs is their low potency and relatively short shelf-life. As soon as one powders an herb, it begins to oxidize and lose its potency. In general, powdered bulk herbs have a shelf-life of only a year or so.

Powdered extracts are the other type of powder and, in fact, are the most commonly used form of ready-made powdered Chinese herbal medicines in the West. These powders are made by the same dual water and alcohol extract method described above. The extract is then either freeze-dried without any fillers or heat dried after being sprayed on some filler. These extracts can be either of single ingredients or entire formulas. Because certain Chinese medicinals can only be extracted to certain potencies, powdered extracts without fillers tend to be different potencies from 5:1 to 20:1 extract ratios. When fillers are used, this is in order to standardize the potencies, typically to the lowest common denominator, *i.e.*, 5:1. Practitioners can either dispense ready-made powdered extract formulas or may create their own, individualized formulas if they have a dispensary of powdered extract singles. A certain amount of these powdered extracts are dissolved in boiling water by the patient each time they take a dose. These powdered extracts are higher potency than pills and bulk powdered herbs. They have a shelf-life if unopened of three years and, if opened, of one year. They are susceptible to damage by exposure to dampness. Their dosage should be calculated on an individual basis taking into account age, weight, condition (whether acute or chronic), severity of symptoms, *and* extract potency. Using high-potency powdered extracts, it is possible to achieve near-decoction potencies in a cost-effective way. However, this depends on the cost of the extracts to the dispensary and the dispensary's mark-up.

Tinctures
Tinctures are made by steeping or soaking bulk Chinese medicinals in alcohol for from two weeks to several months.

Tinctures may be made of either Chinese herbal singles or whole formulas. Traditionally, tinctures were used in Asia by elderly patients taking supplements and anti-rheumatics mainly during the winter months. Tinctures store indefinitely and are easy to dose and take. However, some patients react poorly to alcohol. While it is possible to have a singles pharmacy made up of tinctures, such pharmacies tend to take up a lot of space and all the glass bottles may be expensive. Ready-made Chinese herbal tinctures are more commonly used as external liniments for injuries and rheumatic complaints than for internal administration.

Conclusion

The point of this chapter is that there are different forms of Chinese medicinals and each of these forms has its own benefits and drawbacks. These different forms are not necessarily interchangeable. Dosages need to be carefully considered and adjusted when comparing decoctions to extract powders (with their varying potencies) to low-potency pills. In order to do this, we have to know how the ready-made medicine was made and what the concentration ratio is. This means that practitioners or clinic managers must ask their suppliers about these things if it is not obvious from the information on the packaging. Further, a practitioner or clinic may want to have a dispensary stocked with two or more different forms of medicines. For instance, you might have a bulk pharmacy for the remedial treatment of acute conditions and other seriously ill patients with multi-pattern presentations at the same time as a selection of low-potency pills or higher potency tablets or capsules. Or you might want a singles pharmacy made from low-potency extracts and a number of ready-made formulas in the form of higher potency capsules. What combination of these various forms of Chinese herbal medicines you choose will depend on your training, style of practice, clinic space and employees, and patient population. In other words, there is no "one size fits all" solution.

Problem Based Learning Exercises (See App. IV for answers)

1. In Asia, non-extract powders were traditionally used for emergency situations. Why?

2. Which do you think are more cost-effective for your patients at the same dose equivalencies, bulk-dispensed, water-based decoctions or extract powders? Why? What factors go into answering this question?

3. For the treatment of active disease, most patients will need to (A) increase or (B) decrease the number of Chinese herbal pills they take compared to what is recommended on the typical packaging. Why?

4. Are all powdered extracts equally potent? If not, why not?

5. What is the difference in manufacture between non-extract and extract powders? Which tends to be more potent?

6. What is one drawback of powdered extracts compared to bulk-dispensed, water-based decoctions? What is one benefit of powdered extracts in comparison to bulk-dispensed, water-based decoctions?

7. In determining what form of Chinese herbal medicine to use with a particular patient, you will need to think about the cost-benefit ratio. What is this ratio and how does one use it to solve this problem? Give a concrete example.

8. Your patient needs to take a low dose of Chinese herbal medicines over a very prolonged period of time. In this case, do you think you should prescribe these medicinals in decoction or in pill form? Why? What effect do you think the form of the medicine will have on your patient's compliance?

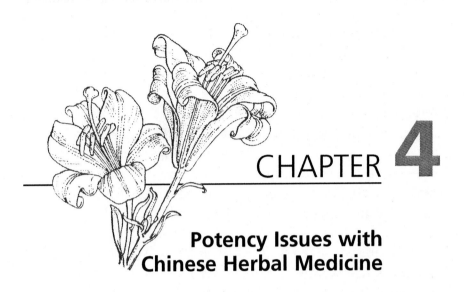

CHAPTER 4

Potency Issues with Chinese Herbal Medicine

Potency is a real issue within Chinese medicine, and by "issue," I mean a problem. One of the criticisms of modern Western medical practitioners of Chinese medicine is that potency is not standardized. In Western medicine, it is assumed that one patient receiving 5mcg of liothyronine (Cytomel®) for hypothyroidism is getting the same dose of medicine as another patient also receiving 5mcg of liothyronine. In Chinese medicine, whether it is with bulk-dispensed, water-based decoctions or even pills and powders, we cannot make the same assumption.

First, let's begin with the bulk herbs themselves. The same species of a particular herb may have more or less active ingredients depending on where the herb was grown, the soil, water, air, sunlight, number of days from planting to harvest, etc. It may also have more or less active ingredients depending on when and how the herb was harvested, dried or otherwise prepared, and the length of time and under what conditions it has been stored. If you have purchased and worked with bulk Chinese herbs, you will know that there are different qualities and that one pound from one supplier does not equal one pound from another supplier in terms of therapeutic effect. If the patient is doing the decoction at home, there are also a number of variables that may effect the therapeutic potency of the decoction. These include the type of cooking vessel used, the amount of water used, whether the herbs were soaked first or not, the temperature of the stove, the cooking times of the individual ingredients, the storage container, refrigeration, and the length of time stored. This means that a patient taking a bulk-dispensed decoction is typically not getting the exact same dosage of medicinals each time, and this may or may not be a problem.

When taking ready-made Chinese herbal pills, tablets, or capsules, although we can assume that a single product from a single manufacturer is the same potency from batch to batch and, therefore, from dose to dose, we cannot assume that the potency is the same for a given formula from manufacturer to manufacturer. In other words, eight pills per time, three times per day of *Xiao Yao Wan* (Rambling Pills) from one manufacturer may not equal the potency of eight pills of *Xiao Yao Wan* from another manufacturer. One manufacturer may use a better quality of raw material than another. Unfortunately, there is little way for the consumer to know what grade or quality raw material their supplier is using. In this case, we must rely on the reputation of the company for quality control at this level.

However, more importantly, one company may manufacture to a different extract ratio than another. When it comes to ready-made Chinese herbal medicines, one of the only ways of identifying comparative potencies is to know the extract ratios. This is definitely knowable with some companies. Another way would be to know the actual weights of specific active ingredients. However, while this method has been used in the nutraceutical industry for herbal supplements, it has not yet been adopted by the ready-made Chinese medicine industry.

Extract ratios

The extract ratio is a description of how much of the raw

material was used to make a given extract. When it comes to ready-made Chinese medicines, these extract ratios can range from 1:1 to 20:1 or more. An extract ratio of 1:1 means that one pound of raw materials was used to make one pound of finished medicine. That means that if one takes three grams of that finished material, one has taken the equivalent of three grams of bulk herbs. A 5:1 extract ratio means that five pounds of raw materials was used to make one pound of finished material. In that case, three grams of that finished product equals 15 grams of bulk herbs. Similarly, a 10:1 extract ratio means that 10 pounds of raw materials were used to make one pound of finished medicine. Therefore, three grams of that medicine equals 30 grams of bulk herbs. In other words, it is assumed that the higher the extract ratio, the more potent is the ready-made medicine.

Most standardized ready-made Chinese medicinal extract powders, whether singles or formulas, are 5:1 extracts. (As of this writing, one company makes standardized 7:1 extract powdered formulas and another company makes standardized powdered extract formulas from 8:1 to 15:1.) It is possible to buy powdered extracts of single medicinals that are higher than this extract ratio. However, such higher potency powdered extract singles are all different extract ratios. For instance, *Huang Qi* (Radix Astragali Membranacei) and *Dang Shen* (Radix Codonopsitis Pilosulae) may be 10:1, *Dang Gui* (Radix Angelicae Sinensis) may be 8:1, but *Da Zao* (Fructus Zizyphi Jujubae) may only be 5:1. This difference has to do with inherent qualities within each herb which only allow it to be extracted singly to certain potencies. As an extension of this, when extracting whole formulas, one can only extract to the limit of the least extractable ingredient.

The Chinese medical yardstick

The professional standard of care in the remedial treatment of disease with Chinese herbal medicines is the bulk-dispensed, water-based decoction discussed in the first chapter of this book. The average standard daily dose of a single Chinese medicinal within a formula administered by this method is 9-10 grams. Knowing this, one can use this number as a yardstick for how potent any dose or any given ready-made Chinese medicine is. For instance, say the ideal formula you would like to write has 15 ingredients in it at an average of 10 grams per ingredient. That means the formula would consist of 150 grams of bulk materials prior to decoction.

Unfortunately, your patient will not take a bulk-dispensed, water-based decoction, so you must prescribe the same formula as an individually made powdered extract formula. Your supplier makes 5:1 powdered extract singles. That means that three grams of this powdered formula equals only 15 grams of bulk medicinals and that is only 1/10 of the standard daily dose for the remedial treatment of disease. Either this dose is likely to be too little to achieve any significant effect or it may achieve an effect but take a very long time to do so. In that case, we can either increase the

> **In our experience, many therapeutic failures among patients of Western practitioners of Chinese medicine are due to insufficient dosage as a result of low-potency ready-made medicines.**

dosage of the original powdered extract or switch to a higher potency extract (if one exists).

In our experience, many therapeutic failures among patients of Western practitioners of Chinese medicine are due to insufficient dosage as a result of low-potency ready-made medicines. The formula was correctly chosen for the patient's pattern and disease, but the dosage administered was way too low.

While standard Chinese dosages may be unnecessarily high if the patient is also receiving acupuncture-moxibustion and Chinese dietary therapy, if the dose is not close to the equivalent of half the standard Chinese daily dose we should not expect too much too soon. That would mean the equivalent of 60-100 grams of bulk Chinese medicinals. As an example, you can easily achieve a dosage equivalency of 90 grams per day of bulk Chinese herbs by taking a 15:1 formula. In that case, one only needs to take six grams of that formula per day to get the equivalent of 90 grams (15 x 6 = 90).

How Many Capsules?
If one capsule contains 500mg by weight (standard in the trade) and you want your patient to take 45, 60 or 75g per day, how many capsules do you need to prescribe?

EXACT RATIO	45G OF MEDICINE	60G OF MEDICINE	75G OF MEDICINE
5:1	18 capsules	24 capsules	30 capsules
6:1	15 capsules	20 capsules	25 capsules
7:1	13 capsules	17 capsules	21 capsules
8:1	11-12 capsules	15 capsules	18 capsules
9:1	10 capsules	13-14 capsules	17 capsules
10:1	9 capsules	12 capsules	15 capsules
12:1	7-8 capsules	10 capsules	12-13 capsules

Note: Anecdotal reports from practitioners in the U.S. suggest that powder extract formulas are well absorbed and may be effective at somewhat lower doses than bulk decoctions. For example, if a bulk decoction comes to 150 grams of dried material, you may be able to get an equal effect with half as much extracted powder. This may be because the manufacturer's extraction process is far more efficient than cooking herbs on a stove and drinking the cooked liquid which is, in fact, not the full 150 grams of ingredients, but a liquid "extraction" of those ingredients in any case.

All this means that it is extremely important to know the extract ratios of any ready-made Chinese medicines you may be using. Until or unless we know these ratios, we have no way of determining the potency of the medicine you are prescribing. Therefore, if this ratio is not clearly stated on the packaging, we have to contact our supplier for this information. If the customer service person on the other end of the phone cannot or will not share this information, it is my advice to run (don't walk) away. Without this information, we are shooting in the dark when it comes to realistically figuring appropriate dosages.

Problem Based Learning Exercises (See App. IV for answers)

1. One powdered extract formula is a 5:1 extract. Another is a 7:1 extract. You want to give your patient the equivalent of 150 grams per day in decoction of a powdered extract. Please compute the number of grams per day necessary to achieve this equivalency with both extracts.

2. You've decided that you are going to give X-number of grams per day of a particular formula in powdered extract form. However, you want to give the patient a strong dose of additional *Huang Qi* (Radix Astragali Membranacei). One of your suppliers carries a 12:1 extract of *Huang Qi*. How many grams of this extract do you need to prescribe per day of this *Huang Qi* in order to equal 30 grams per day in decoction?

3. Your supplier has told you that you should typically prescribe six grams of their powdered extract per day and that they are 5:1 extracts. However, you have read that the same formula is typically prescribed at a dosage of 200 grams per day in decoction in China for the same pattern of the same disease and that 75% of patients responded positively to that dosage in two weeks. Your patient is not seeing the results she would like to, and she is getting impatient with your care. What do you do and why?

4. Currently, the Chinese herbal profession does not use standardized extracts of specific active ingredients. Why do you think this is? Can you think of at least one reason not to use such standardized extracts of active ingredients derived from parts of Chinese medicinals? For instance, pentosan is an active chemical ingredient in *Tong Cao* (Medulla Tetrapanacis Papyriferi). Why not just use pentosan instead of *Tong Cao*?

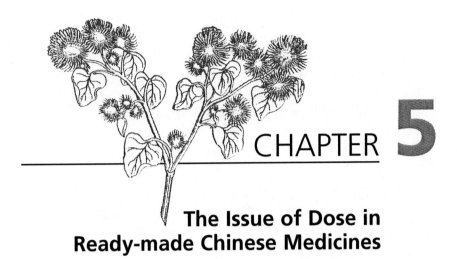

CHAPTER 5

The Issue of Dose in Ready-made Chinese Medicines

If you are like me, you get at least one spam per day offering Western prescription drugs either at a discount or without a doctor's prescription. If you have ever looked at any of these offers, you know that any given Western prescription medicine and even many over-the-counter [OTC] medicines typically come in a variety of dosages. For example, the antidepressant amitriptyline (Elavil) comes in 10, 25, 50, 75, 100, and 150mg tablets. The antianxiety medicine alprozolam (Xanax) comes in 0.25, 0.5, 1, and 2mg tablets. The beta-blocker atenolol (Tenormin) comes in 25, 50, and 100mg tablets, and levothyroxine (L-Thyroxine) comes in 0.0125, 0.025, 0.037, 0.05, 0.075, 0.088, 0.1, 0.112, 0.125, 0.15, 0.175, 0.2, and 0.3mg tablets. This variety of dosages for the same medicine underscores a fact that any Western MD knows: different patients may need different dosages of the same medicine.

In China, ready-made medicines (usually in low-dose pill form) are rarely prescribed by professional Chinese medical practitioners. They are primarily meant for A) over-the-counter use by laypersons and B) the treatment of chronic conditions and/or C) the consolidation of therapeutic results after more active remedial therapy. Therefore, the stated dosages on their packaging tend to be very low to prevent accidental overdose by the untrained. The problem is that, here in the West, many professional practitioners do prescribe these kinds of ready-made Chinese medicines for the remedial treatment of an active disease. However, in my experience, many patients are simply told to take the dosage written on the label. Often times that is what we were taught in school and, after all, those are the directions, aren't they?

The answer to that question is both yes and no. Yes if the person is buying the medicine OTC on their own volition. No if I am prescribing the medicine professionally to one of my patients for the remedial treatment of an active disease. In that case, as a prescribing physician (no matter what my legal title), it is my responsibility to determine exactly what dosage is the best for each individual patient. Just as one dose of Western pharmaceuticals does not fit all, so also a single dose of Chinese medicinals does not fit everyone. In fact, the determination of correct dose is one of the things our patients are paying us for whether they know it or not. So, what are some of the criteria necessary for us to determine the correct dose of a Chinese ready-made medicine?

Five Criteria to Determine the Correct Dose
- **age**
- **weight**
- **disease severity**
- **disease diagnosis**
- **medicinal strength**

There are five things to keep in mind when trying to determine the correct dose for a given patient: 1) age, 2) weight, 3) disease severity, 4) disease diagnosis, and 5) medicinal strength. For instance, babies and young children should be given smaller doses than adults due, in part, to their immature metabolisms and medicinal sensitivity. However, the elderly (*i.e.*, those over 60) should also receive half doses due to the decline in function of the digestive system as well as the liver and kidneys. Because the elderly do not metabolize medicines as quickly as younger adults do, medicines stay in their systems longer. The second thing to take into account is a patient's weight or body mass. The larger the patient's body, the more medicine they typically will require to catalyze changes in that mass of cells. That means a patient who weighs 300 pounds will require significantly more medicine than a patient who weighs 150. Below are tables presenting standard guidelines of dosing according to age and weight.

AGE-TO-DOSE GUIDELINES

0-1 month	1/18-1/14 of adult dose
1-6 months	1/14-1/7 of adult dose
6-12 months	1/7-1/5 of adult dose
1-2 years	1/5-1/4 of adult dose
2-4 years	1/4-1/3 of adult dose
4-6 years	1/3-2/5 of adult dose
6-9 years	2/5-1/2 of adult dose
9-14 years	1/2-2/3 of adult dose
14-18 years	2/3 to full adult dose
18-60 years	full adult dose
60 years +	3/4 adult dose or less

WEIGHT-TO-DOSE GUIDELINES

30-40 lbs.	20-27% of adult dose
40-50 lbs.	27-33% of adult dose
50-60 lbs.	33-40% of adult dose
60-70 lbs.	40-47% of adult dose
70-80 lbs.	47-53% of adult dose
80-100 lbs.	53-67% of adult dose
100-120 lbs.	67-80% of adult dose
120-150 lbs.	80-100% of adult dose
150-200 lbs.	100-133% of adult dose
200-250 lbs.	133-167% of adult dose
250-300 lbs.	167-200% of adult dose

Patients who are more than usually sensitive to foods, herbs, or drugs should begin with smaller than usual doses.

The third factor is disease severity. In Chinese medicine, the more severe or acute a disease, the higher the doses we usually administer. That is because we are trying to achieve results as quickly as possible in order to minimize pain and suffering as well as the possibility of irreversible damage.

The fourth factor is the disease diagnosis. The disease diagnosis tells us the natural history of the condition, for instance, whether it is self-limiting, relapsing-remittent, chronic, progressive, disabling, fatal, etc. In acute diseases of expected short duration, we typically prescribe high doses to knock the disease out as quickly as possible, while, in chronic, lingering, slowly progressive diseases, we typically prescribe lower doses in a more user-friendly form of administration so that we can assure good patient adherence over a long period of time. For example, in a relapsing-remittent disease such as MS, we may prescribe high dose decoctions during relapses and low dose ready-made medicines during remittent stages.

The fifth factor in determining dosage is somewhat more difficult to deal with at the moment due to some companies not transparently telling practitioners how to assess the strength of their medicines. As stated above, without knowing how strong a medicine is, how can we determine what its dose should be? Perhaps, since practitioners have not asked for this information, these companies have not figured there is a need for it. However, if we ever intend to earn the status, respect, and earnings of Western MDs, we must eventually practice medicine, albeit Chinese medicine, at the same professional level, and that means prescribing individualized dosages of medicines to individual patients. Therefore, one of the first questions when considering prescribing a Chinese ready-made medicine to a patient is, "How strong is that medicine?"

Since most Chinese ready-made medicines are made from extracts, one way of answering that question is to know the concentration ratio used in making that medicine. If a medicine is a 5:1 extract, that means that five pounds of bulk herbs were used to make one pound of finished medicine. If it is a 7:1 extract, it means that seven pounds of bulk herbs were used to make one pound of finished medicine, and, if it is a 12:1 extract, it means that 12 pounds of bulk herbs were used to make one pound of finished medicine. The assumption here is that the higher the concentration ratio, the more potent the medicine.

However, that still does not tell us everything we need to know. In standard professional Chinese medicine, the average daily dose of a single medicinal is nine grams (9g). If there are 10 ingredients in a formula, that means a dose of 90 grams per day made into decoction. If we want our patient to receive the equivalent of not less than 90 grams of Chinese medicinals per day for the remedial treatment of active disease, then we would need to prescribe 18 grams per day of a 5:1 extract, 12.6 grams per day of a 7:1 extract, nine grams per day of a 10:1 extract, and only six grams per day of a 15:1 extract. In real life, if a patient is also receiving acupuncture, they might not need the equivalent of 90 grams per day since, unlike in China, they are being treated by more than one modality. So maybe we could cut the dose down to 60 or even 45g per day. In that case, it would only take nine grams per day of a 5:1 extract, 4.5 grams per day of a 10:1 extract, and three grams per day of a 15:1 extract. (See chart on p. 75)

Since, typically, unwanted side effects are directly proportional to increased dose, in general as prescribing physicians, we want the lowest dose which will achieve the intended therapeutic effects within the desired timeframe. This also means

> . . .if you're not getting the results you expect from Chinese ready-made medicines, A) raise the dose and B) consider using a higher concentration extract.

starting patients with chronic diseases with low doses and then raising those doses, increment by increment, until one achieves the intended therapeutic effect with either no or the least adverse reactions. In closing, if you're not getting the results you expect from Chinese ready-made medicines, A) raise the dose and B) consider using a higher concentration extract.

Final note: For those of you who treat infants and young children, the question commonly arises as to the best way to administer Chinese medicine to our young patients. First of all, very young children may be less resistant that you presume to taking decocted Chinese medicine. We suggest the easiest way to administer it is to use an eye-dropper, giving 1-2 droppers between 3-8 times per day, depending upon the severity of the child's condition. This is easier than dealing with pills or capsules, which small children often cannot swallow. For breast-feeding infants, it is also acceptable to create a paste from extract powders and rub a small amount on the mother's nipple, administering with the breast milk.

Problem Based Learning Exercises (See App. IV for answers)

1. Two patients present the same patterns suggesting that they should take the same Chinese herbal formula. One patient is a 45 year-old male of medium build. You decided that he should take a decoction made from a total of 150 grams of Chinese medicinals per day. The other patient is a six year-old child. Using standard age dosing guidelines, what should be the total daily dose of Chinese medicinals expressed in grams?
2. Another two patients present the same patterns suggesting once again that they should both take the same Chinese herbal formula. The patients are both middle-aged adults. However, one weighs 160 pounds and the other weighs 240 pounds. You decided to give the 160-pound patient a daily dose of six grams of powdered extract per day. Based on weight differential alone, how many grams should you give per day to the 240-pound patient?

3. *Dao Chi San* (Abduct the Red Powder) is for the treatment of heart-small intestine fire causing heart palpitations, vexation, agitation, and restlessness, sores on the tip of the tongue, and short, scanty, difficult, burning, and painful urination with dark-colored urine or hematuria.

    A. Is this an acute or chronic condition?

    B. Based on the above answer, what should be the daily dose of this formula when given in decoction?

4. *Liu Wei Di Huang Wan* (Six Flavors Rehmannia Pills) and *Bu Zhong Yi Qi Tang* (Supplement the Center & Boost the Qi Pills) are given to a patient with a tendency to high blood glucose presenting with qi and yin dual vacuity and liver depression qi stagnation in order to secure and consolidate the treatment effects from more aggressive remedial therapy. At the moment, the patient's blood sugar is within normal limits, but you don't want the patient to regress. How are you going to decide how many of each pills to advise the patient to take?

5. Your patient refuses to drink bulk-dispensed, water-based decoctions because they taste bad, smell up her house, and take too long to cook. You've decided that she needs to take the equivalent of 200 grams per day of bulk-dispensed herbs based on the severity and nature of her condition. She will, however, take powdered extracts and you have the same formula from a company that makes 5:1 extracts. How many grams of this extract must the patient take per day in order to get the equivalent of 200 grams of bulk medicinals in decoction?

6. Your patient has an acute earache due to liver fire flaming upward and you want him to take at least 2-3 days' worth of *Long Dan Xie Gan Tang* (Gentiana Drain the Liver Decoction) in decoction form. How are you going to explain to him the necessity/benefits of taking his Chinese medicinals in this form?

7. What are the standard daily doses in decoction given in Bensky & Gamble for the following commonly used medicinals:

    A. *Sha Ren* (Fructus Amomi)

    B. *Pu Gong Ying* (Herba Taraxaci Mongolici Cum Radice)

C. *Bai Jiang Cao* (Herba Patriniae Heterophyllae)
D. *Chai Hu* (Radix Bupleuri)
E. *Ban Xia* (Rhizoma Pinelliae Ternatae)
F. *Huang Qi* (Radix Astragali Membranacei)
G. *Dang Shen* (Radix Codonopsitis Pilosulae)
H. *Chuan Xiong* (Radix Ligustici Wallichii)
I. *Sheng Di* (uncooked Radix Rehmanniae Glutinosae)
J. *Bai Zhu* (Rhizoma Atractylodis Macrocephalae)
K. *Fu Ling* (Sclerotium Poriae Cocos)
L. *Gan Jiang* (dry Rhizoma Zingiberis Officinalis)
M. *Xiang Fu* (Rhizoma Cyperi Rotundi)
N. *Dang Gui* (Radix Angelicae Sinensis)
O. *He Shou Wu* (Radix Polygoni Multiflori)
P. *Ji Xue Teng* (Caulis Milletiae Seu Spatholobi)

8. Your patient with a chronic condition says that she has multiple chemical sensitivities. Do you start her on the standard daily dose? Why?

9. You plan on combining acupuncture and internally administered Chinese herbal medicine with your patient. How does this affect the dose of Chinese herbal medicinals you plan on administering? Why?

10. Why should a patient with coronary artery disease (CAD) and unstable angina pectoris be given a higher dose of Chinese medicinals than a patient with asymptomatic CAD?

11. Why should a patient with rheumatoid arthritis (RA) which is currently in remission be given a lower dose of Chinese medicinals than a patient with active RA?

12. Why should a patient with kidney failure be given a higher dose of Chinese medicinals than a patient with interstitial cystitis?

CHAPTER 6

The Phenomenon of Habituation in Long-term Herbal Treatment

We have all had the experience of "tuning out" a constant noise or smell. When the body receives a constant stimulus, over time, it tends to discount and filter out that stimulus. When the body filters out and discounts the effects of a medicinal substance, this is referred to technically as habituation. Habituation may be defined as the progressive decrease in responsiveness to repetitive stimuli.[1] In modern Western medicine, this is a well known phenomenon. M. Leandri, author of an article titled "Therapy of Trigeminal Neuralgia Secondary to Multiple Sclerosis" published in issue #5, 2003, of *Expert Review of Anticancer Therapy,* in speaking about the medical treatment of trigeminal neuralgia, writes, "Whatever the drug, habituation and loss of efficacy are likely to occur sooner or later."[2] In discussing what to do about this phenomenon, Leandri goes on to say:

> Dosage should be as low as possible for the risk of habituation . . . and therapy should be slowly tapered off from time to time. When forced to increase dosage, always check the neurological conditions, beside the usual biological checks as indicated. If side effects appear, cautiously switch to another compound . . .[3]

[1] http://ericfacility.net/extra/newauth/thesfull.cfm?TERM=Habituation
[2] www.future-drugs.com/summery.asp?articleid=925&submit=txt2
[3] *Ibid.*

What many North American practitioners of Chinese medicine may not realize is that this same process affects our prescription of, and our patients' response to, Chinese herbal medicine. While numerous herbal medicine Websites parrot the following erroneous party line,

> Botanical nervines, on the other hand, are free from toxicity and habituation. Because they are organic substances and not man-made synthetic molecules, they possess a natural affinity for the human organism . . .[4]

This is just not true in my experience. Every now and again, a practitioner will call Blue Poppy's help line with the following observations and questions. When they first started a particular patient or patients on a Blue Poppy Herbs formula, the results were immediate and dramatic. However, after prolonged usage, the formula does not seem to be getting the same response. Therefore, have we changed the formula to make it less effective? In this situation, our customer service representatives always check with production to make sure that the formula is still being manufactured in exactly the same way, with the same ingredients and dosages, by the same manufacturer. If, in fact, this is the case, commonly what we find is that the practitioner has had the patient on the same formula at the same dose for months at a time without a break.

> **In China, both acupuncture and Chinese herbal practitioners are well aware of the phenomenon of habituation.**

In China, both acupuncture and Chinese herbal practitioners are well aware of the phenomenon of habituation. Typically, for chronic conditions, acupuncture patients receive multiple courses of treatment. Those courses may be a week long, 10 days long, or a month long (as in many gynecological conditions associated with irregularities of the menstrual cycle). Patients receive either a treatment every day or every other day. At the end of

---

[4] www.shirleys-wellness-cafe.com/nervines.htm

each course, there is a scheduled break. For instance, there may be a one- or two-day break every week if the patient is receiving weekly courses of five or six treatments. Or there may be a break of a 2-7 days when courses are longer. In the case of gynecological complaints, frequently the rest periods are the menses themselves which may last anywhere from 3-7 days. Likewise, when patients are taking the same Chinese medicinal formula day in and day out for prolonged periods of time, they are allowed to take periodic breaks. Since internal medicine courses of treatment tend to be longer in duration, two weeks to a month or longer in most cases, these breaks tend to last 5-7 days.

These breaks or rest periods are a vitally important part of long-term therapy for chronic, enduring diseases. They allow the patient's physiology to desensitize itself to the medicinal stimuli so that when the acupuncture or administration of internal Chinese herbal medicine is resumed, it will have

> . . . as practitioners, we are (or at least should be) always looking for the best therapeutic effect at the lowest possible dose, and periodic rests are one way of achieving that goal.

renewed effect without necessarily having to increase the dosages. As we all know, the tendency to producing adverse medicinal reactions is commonly dose-dependent. This means that adverse reactions (or so-called side effects) tend to occur more frequently the higher the dose of the medicinal. This is true for Chinese herbal medicinals as well. Therefore, as practitioners, we are (or at least should be) always looking for the best therapeutic effect at the lowest possible dose, and periodic rests are one way of achieving that goal. Without such regularly scheduled breaks in treatment, our patients will become desensitized and habituated to their Chinese herbal medicine with the result that both we and they will see progressively diminishing returns.

When treating women with gynecological complaints that do

not pathologically affect the flow of blood of the menses itself, it is always a good idea to stop treatment during menstruation. The main exceptions to this are dysmenorrhea and excessively profuse menstruation (*i.e.*, menorrhagia). Likewise, treatment may be suspended during menstruation in women who are being treated for non-gynecological complaints. Men do not typically have such an obvious monthly cycle. Nevertheless, they too should undergo periodic rests from treatment. Either these rests can be two or more days per month or 6-7 days every six weeks to two months. However, no matter what schedule you choose, periodic rests in treatment are usually extremely important when therapy stretches over months and months as in the case of conditions such as high cholesterol, benign prostatic hypertrophy (BPH), multiple sclerosis (MS), rheumatoid arthritis (RA), systemic lupus erythmatosus (SLE), psoriasis, and hypertension. So if you have noticed diminishing returns and are not regularly scheduling periodic breaks in therapy, this is something I strongly advise you to consider.

Case History Exercises (See App. IV for answers)

Case: Male, 32 years old

Your patient has been receiving treatment for recurrent right-sided lower abdominal pain for several months. This man came to you because, after every test in the book, Western MDs failed to identify any reason for his abdominal pain. So the man decided to try an alternative approach. The Chinese herbal medicine you prescribed for this patient was extremely effective. However, after taking it for six months at a consistent dose, the patient has called to say that it doesn't seem to be working as effectively any longer.
1. What do you do first?
2. What questions might you ask the man?
3. If you have ruled out any changes in diet, exercise, work,

lifestyle, etc. that might be negating the effect of the remedy prescribed, what is the next thing to consider?

4. How are you going to confirm or deny this hypothesis?

5. If it turns out that the patient's pattern remains basically the same, what are you going to suggest? Up the dosage or take a few days off the medicine? Why?

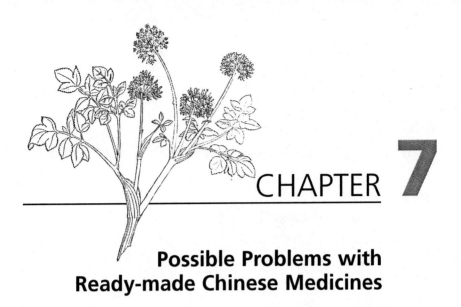

CHAPTER **7**

Possible Problems with Ready-made Chinese Medicines

There are several potential problems with ready-made Chinese medicines in terms of quality control. These primarily have to do with contamination, adulteration, and mislabeling.

Contamination

Contamination of ready-made Chinese medicinals can be due to heavy metals, pesticides, and microbes. While heavy metal contamination potentially affects all commercially grown Chinese herbal medicinals, both bulk and ready-made, due to the concentration processes by which most ready-made Chinese medicines are made, these processes can also concentrate heavy metals in the finished product. As part of their "feeding" on the soil in which they live, plants take up heavy metals from the ground in which they are grown and from the water which they "drink." Some soils, due to use of certain pesticides and fertilizers contain more heavy metals than others. Likewise, certain bodies of water contain higher concentrations of heavy metals due to their proximity to manufacturing facilities which release heavy metals into the air and thence enter the water. In addition, heavy metals can enter a ready-made medicine in the manufacturing process itself if, for instance the factory uses lead solder in its manufacturing equipment or plumbing.

The heavy metals that are especially of concern in terms of human toxicity are arsenic, cadmium, chromium, lead and mercury. While it is very difficult to completely and absolutely eliminate all traces of these heavy metals from Chinese medicinals, through proper manufacturing processes, they can be rendered so small (in terms of parts per million) that their impact on the human body is virtually inconsequential. Therefore, our suggestion is to only buy ready-made Chinese medicinals from companies who test their medicines for heavy metal contamination and are willing to share with their customers and the public the results of those tests.

> **While it is very difficult to completely and absolutely eliminate all traces of these heavy metals from Chinese medicinals, through proper manufacturing processes, they can be rendered so small (in terms of parts per million) that their impact on the human body is virtually inconsequential.**

When vegetable crops, including medicinal herbs, are grown commercially, pesticides which are harmful to human health, may be picked up by these herbs. There are two main types of pesticides which may be harmful to human health. These are called organophosphate pesticides and chlorinated pesticides. Some well-known toxic organophosphate pesticides include Dursban®, Guthion®, Roneet®, Co Ral®, Naled®, Nemacur®, Phosmet®, and Rubitox®. Examples of well-known but potentially harmful chlorinated pesticides include 4,4 DDD, 4,4 DDT, 4,4 DDE, BHC-A, BHC-B, BHC-D, BHC-G, Captan®, Chlordane®, Endrin®, Pyrethrum®, Dylox®, and Mavrik®. One way to avoid contamination by pesticides is to use organically grown Chinese herbs. However, this industry, while growing, is in its infancy in China and other countries supplying Chinese medicinal herbs. It is also possible to reduce the amounts of pesticides through "washing" processes during manufacture. Therefore, we also recommend that you ask your Chinese herbal suppliers for copies of tests analyzing the concentra-

94

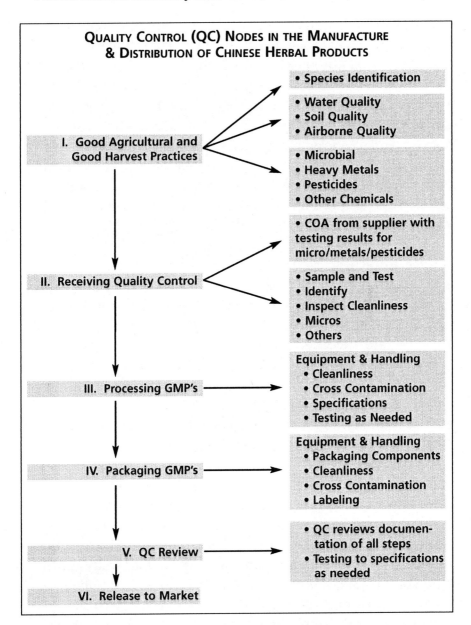

QUALITY CONTROL (QC) NODES IN THE MANUFACTURE
& DISTRIBUTION OF CHINESE HERBAL PRODUCTS

I. Good Agricultural and Good Harvest Practices
- Species Identification
- Water Quality
- Soil Quality
- Airborne Quality
- Microbial
- Heavy Metals
- Pesticides
- Other Chemicals

II. Receiving Quality Control
- COA from supplier with testing results for micro/metals/pesticides
- Sample and Test
- Identify
- Inspect Cleanliness
- Micros
- Others

III. Processing GMP's
Equipment & Handling
- Cleanliness
- Cross Contamination
- Specifications
- Testing as Needed

IV. Packaging GMP's
Equipment & Handling
- Packaging Components
- Cleanliness
- Cross Contamination
- Labeling

V. QC Review
- QC reviews documentation of all steps
- Testing to specifications as needed

VI. Release to Market

tions of both organophosphate pesticides and chlorinated pesticides in their products. Testing should be done for approximately 200 pesticides known to be harmful to humans. (See Appendix V).

The third type of contamination of ready-made Chinese medicinals is microbial. Microbial contamination describes potential human toxicity due to the presence of unacceptably high number of pathogenic organisms in the medicinal. The two main classes of microbes which may contaminate ready-made Chinese medicinals are bacteria and yeast and molds. The main pathogenic bacteria, that should be routinely tested for by manufacturers of ready-made Chinese medicinals are *Salmonella, Escherichia coli, Klebsiella, Serratia, Staphylococcus aureus,* and *Bacillus sp.* as well as the total of all species of bacteria present in the finished product. The main types of pathogenic yeast and molds which should be tested for are *Aspergillus niger* and *Candida albicans.*

Adulteration

Adulteration in the manufacture of Chinese ready-made medicinals means the addition of Western pharmaceuticals to a traditional Chinese herbal formula in order to make it more powerful and effective. The following is a list of some adulterants that have been found in certain Chinese ready-made, supposedly herbal medicines: acetaminophen, aminopyrine, chlorpheniramine, chlorzoxazone, phenacetin, and phenylbutazone. Some of these are over-the-counter medications in the West and some are by-prescription-only. Some have been taken off the market in the U.S. due to reports of toxicity, including death. While the Ministry of Health in the People's Republic of China have made it illegal to manufacture Chinese herbal medicines adulterated by Western pharmaceuticals, companies operating outside the PRC are still engaging in this practice. Therefore, it is important to buy ready-made Chinese medicinals only from well-established, reputable, and transparent companies. Customers should feel free to ask their suppliers for certificates of analysis (COA) documenting exactly what is in each and every medicine.

Mislabeling

While not as much of a problem as in the past, mislabeling can also cause toxic reactions. Mislabeling here refers to the incomplete disclosure of ingredients, improper listing of ingredients, and/or the misidentification of ingredients. In the past, many Asian firms sought to keep their proprietary formulas secret by failing to completely disclose all the ingredients in a product. Without knowing all the ingredients in a product, there is no way for a practitioner to rationally assess the probabilities of a toxic reaction in a particular individual. It has also been common for Asians to misidentify the ingredients in their products simply through ignorance of either Pinyin or Western pharmacognosy and Latin pharmacological nomenclature. This sometimes means that the ingredients are correctly identified in Chinese (in Chinese characters) but incorrectly identified in either Pinyin or Latin. Just as it is impossible to rationally judge the probability of a toxic reaction if one does not know all the ingredients, neither can one make such a determination if the ingredients contained are not the ones that are listed.

> **Over the past several years, there have been great improvements in the labeling of ready-made Chinese medicinals for sale in the U.S.**

Over the past several years, there have been great improvements in the labeling of ready-made Chinese medicinals for sale in the U.S. Basically, all companies selling herbal supplements in the U.S. must follow the Food & Drug Administration (FDA)'s food labeling rules. This means that all ingredients must be disclosed, beginning with the ingredient in largest proportion by weight to the ingredient in smallest proportion by weight. There must be a supplement fact panel as well as a serving size. And finally, there must also be instructions for use.

Unfortunately, when it comes to instructions for use, the FDA does not allow a dosage range but requires a specific daily dose. Because companies are commonly worried about litigation from persons who either accidentally or purposefully take too much, they tend to print low-end doses on their labels.

This means that practitioners must commonly increase the stated dosages on the packaging in order for their patients to achieve the expected therapeutic effects in a timely manner.

Problem Based Learning Exercises (See App. IV for answers)

1. Go on-line and look at the U.S. FDA's rules and regulations governing the labeling of dietary supplements under DSHEA (Dietary Supplement Health Education Act). Then look at the labels of a number of ready-made Chinese medicines from various sources (*i.e.*, from various companies in different parts of Asia as well as from North American and/or European companies). Then answer the following questions:

A. Do these labels conform to U.S. FDA rules and regulations?

B. Do the herbal medicinal identifications seem to be correct for each formula based on what you know?

2. Ask your Chinese herb supplier(s) to provide you with a certificate of analysis (COA) for each of the above products. Does this/do these COA(s) tally with the ingredients on the label(s)?

3. Ask your Chinese herb supplier(s) to provide you with laboratory reports on heavy metal, pesticide residue, and microbial contamination for each of the above products.

A. Are they willing to do this?

B. Can they do this?

C. Are the laboratory results within safe and acceptable ranges? To answer this last question, you may have to find out what safe and acceptable ranges are.

D. Do/does the supplier(s) test every batch of every formula?

4. Are there batch numbers on the packaging to allow for a recall if necessary?

5. Are there expiration dates?

6. Go on-line to the FDA's Web site and read about ready-made Chinese medicines that have been found to contain adulterants. Are any of these medicines among the ones you are looking at as part of these exercises?

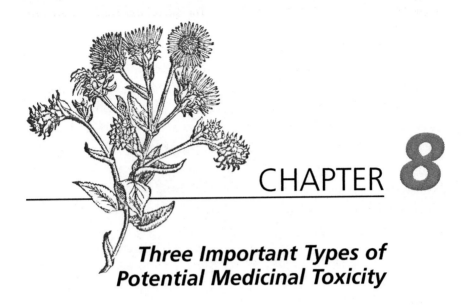

CHAPTER **8**

Three Important Types of Potential Medicinal Toxicity

In the past decade, three types of toxicity have received attention and driven concern over the safety of Chinese medicinal substances. These are nephrotoxicity, hepatotoxicity, and fetotoxicity.

Nephrotoxicity

The greatest concern over the toxicity of Chinese medicinal products remains the potential for nephrotoxicity. This concern was driven by the Belgium incident of the early to mid-90s.[1] The cause of the nephropathy experienced by the women who took the dangerous "slimming formula" was thought to be aristolochic acid, a known nephrotoxin. The medicinal singled out for the nephrotoxicity was *Han Fang Ji* (Radix Stephaniae Tetandrae) which was alleged to be in the capsules consumed by the women.[2] However, subsequent chromatographic examination of the capsules showed that they did not contain the compound tetandrine which is a major compo-

---

[1]Blackwell, Richard, *Cases of Herb Toxicity*, http:/acupuncture.com/herbolo gy/toxic.htm, 1996, p. 1-3

[2]It should be noted that *Han Fang Ji*, while having diuretic qualities, is not commonly used by trained Oriental medicine practitioners for weight loss. It is generally decocted with medicinals such as *Fu Ling* (Sclerotium Poriae Cocos) and *Gui Zhi* (Ramulus Cinnamomi Cassiae) to treat lower body edema due to fluid accumulation.

nent of *Han Fang Ji* and is used as a chemical marker for this medicinal. Later research suggested that the aristolochic acid intoxication might have come from a different source, such as the medicinal *Guang Fang Ji* (Radix Aristolochia Fangji) which does contain aristolochic acid and may have been included in the capsules due to a purchasing and identification error by the practitioners prescribing it. Or else the toxicity originated from a combination of other causes, such as the low carbohydrate diet the patients were on which might have accelerated and enhanced the effect of all the pharmaceutical products in the formula. It may have also been due to the fact that the Chinese medicinals were not prepared in a decoction but ground up raw, thus greatly increasing their individual potency. Another possibility is that the toxicity resulted from the strange combination of medicinals which included Western appetite inhibitors, including the now banned pharmaceutical, fenfluramine.

> *Regardless of the cause, upon hearing of the reports from Belgium, the FDA branded all Chinese medicinals containing even trace amounts of aristolochic acid before cooking as being toxic and began moving to prohibit their sale and prescription by 2001.*

Regardless of the cause, upon hearing of the reports from Belgium, the FDA branded all Chinese medicinals containing even trace amounts of aristolochic acid before cooking as being toxic and began moving to prohibit their sale and prescription by 2001.[3] In addition to *Guang Fang Ji* and *Han Fang Ji*, these substances included *Mu Tong* (Caulis Mutong), *Wei Ling Xian* (Radix Clematidis), and *Xi Xin* (Herba Asari Cum Radice), popular and effective medicinals which appear in many formulas.[4] Despite little evidence that these medicinals, when prepared and dosed

---

[3]FDA Consumer Advisory, http://www.cfsan.fda.gov/~dms/addsbot.html
[4]Chen, J., "Aristolochic Acid and Chinese Herbs,"
http://acupuncture.com/Herbology/aristo.htm, p. 1-3

properly, can cause nephropathy, they remain banned today. Fortunately, a number of respected American pharmaceutical companies who manufacture Chinese medicinal formulas have found a way to process these forbidden herbs so that the trace amounts of aristolochic acid they contain are removed prior to decoction, a measure that should solve the potential toxicity problem. In the meantime, most Oriental medical practitioners are either eliminating these medicinals from their formulas or substituting other medicinals with similar actions to take their place.

Hepatotoxicity

In general, the advantage of most Chinese medicinals is that they are quickly processed and passed out of the liver with no hepatoxic effects. However there are some exceptions which should be noted. *Cang Er Zi* (Fructus Xanthii Sibirici), a commonly used herb for many nasal symptoms, can be both hepato- and nephrotoxic if not decocted properly with other medicinals. This is an example of "mutual counteraction,"[5] wherein the toxic medicinal's potentially toxic effects are eliminated by one or more other substances. The potentially toxic effects of many herbs can be eliminated by appropriate herbal preparation.

Another example is the unfortunate result that may occur when some Chinese herbal medicinals interact with orthodox Western drugs in the liver. Just as the combination of acetaminophen (Tylenol®) and alcohol can create a potentially fatal hepatotoxicity, so too can the medicinals *He Zi* (Fructus Terminaliae Chebulae), *Wu Bei Zi* (Galla Rhois Chinensis), or *Di Yu* (Radix Sanguisorbae Officinalis) create a hepatoxic combination when processed in the liver with isoniazid, tetracyclines, rifampcin, chlorpromazine, or erythromycin.[6] Patients taking any of these Western pharmaceuticals should be moni-

---

[5]Bensky, Dan & Gamble, Andrew, *Chinese Medicine: Materia Medica*, Eastland Press, Seattle, 1993, p. 9
[6]Chan, K. & Cheung, L., *Interactions Between Chinese Herbal Medicinal Products and Orthodox Drugs*, Taylor and Francis, London, 2003, p. 72

tored carefully to guard against accidental poisoning due to the combination effects of these substances.

A third example of hepatotoxicity due to Chinese medicinals came as the result of the liver damage caused by a ready-made medicine called *Jin Bu Huan* (More Precious Than Gold), a once-popular remedy for insomnia and pain. In 1993-94, seven adults taking the brand of this formula manufactured by the Kwangsi Pai Se Company developed symptoms of hepatitis consistent with a drug reaction. Although the mechanism that caused the hepatitis in this small number of individuals is still unclear, investigators at the time concluded that it was due to an immunoallergic reaction because of the eosinophilia found in the liver biopsies

> *Over the past several years, there have been great improvements in the labeling of ready-made Chinese medicinals for sale in the U.S.*

of two of the patients. At first, it was thought this was perhaps due to a reaction to its supposed primary ingredient, *Yuan Zhi* (Radix Polygalae Tenuofoliae). However, further investigation found that the alkaloids in the remedy did not match those of the *Polygala* family but rather that of the blood-quickening herb *Yan Hu Suo* (Rhizoma Corydalis Yanhusuo). So it remains uncertain whether the remedy contained the wrong medicinal or was adulterated by some other substance which caused the actual hepatotoxicity.[7] In either case, the result was that *Jin Bu Huan* was banned in the United States and the United Kingdom. Curiously, this is still a popular remedy in Far and Southeast Asia with no reports of hepatotoxicity from its use in those regions. In any case, these immunoallergic reactions in the U.S. were instrumental in focusing attention on the issue of toxicity and Chinese medicinals with subsequent efforts on the part of manufacturers and distributors to substantially increase quality control.

---

[7]Blackwell, *op. cit.*, p. 3-4.

Risk factors predisposing one to hepatotoxicity include:

> - *Previous notable adverse reactions to drugs or herbs*
> - *A history of a number of different allergies*
> - *A history of chronic skin rashes*
> - *Pre-existing liver disease*

Stop signs when using herbs include:

> *1. Development of a substantial skin rash*
>
> *2. Nausea or bloating*
>
> *3. Worsening fatigue*
>
> *4. Aching in the area of the liver, yellowing of the eyes or skin, reduction in coloration of the feces*

Medicinal-induced hepatitis is defined as inflammation of the liver resulting in loss of integrity of the cell membranes causing leakage of cells' contents into blood plasma. Therefore, there is elevation of the liver enzymes AST (a.k.a. SGOP) and ALT (a.k.a. SGOT) when blood testing is performed.

Fetotoxicity

Perhaps the most difficult type of toxicity facing the practitioner of either Western or Oriental medicinal products is the potential for causing fetotoxicity. The developing embryo is so vulnerable to damage caused by foreign substances in the mother's blood stream that many Western and Oriental medicinal products, while quite safe for an adult,

> *Perhaps the most difficult type of toxicity facing the practitioner of either Western or Oriental medicinal products is the potential for causing fetotoxicity.*

are considered problematic and potentially lethal for the fetus, either by direct poisoning or by causing spontaneous abortion.

Some potentially fetotoxic Chinese medicinals include:

Qian Niu Zi (Semen Pharbiditis)
Gan Sui (Radix Euphorbiae Kansui)
Yuan Hua (Flos Daphhis Genkwae)
Jing Da Ji (Radix Euphrobiae Seu Knoxiae)
Shang Lu (Radix Phytolaccae)
Tian Hua Fen (Radix Trichosanthis Kirlowii)
Bai Fu Zi (Rhizoma Typhonii Gigantei Seu Radix
Aconiti Koreani)
Zao Jiao (Fructus Gleditschiae Chinensis)
Zao Jiao Ci (Spina Gleditschiae Chinensis)
Fu Zi (Radix Lateralis Praeparatus Aconiti
Carmichaeli)
Wu Gong (Scolopendra Subspinipes)
Qing Fen (Calomelas)
Xiong Huang (Realgar)
Liu Huang (Sulphur)
Ma Qian Zi (Semen Strychnotis Nux-vomicae)
Mu Bie Zi (Semen Mormordicae Cochinensis)
Zhang Nao (Camphora)
Ban Mao (Mylabris)
Chan Su (Secretio Bufonis)
Kuan Jin Teng (Caulis Tinosporae Sinensis)

For more information of Chinese herbal toxicities and drug interactions, see Fred Jennes' *Herb Toxicities & Drug Interactions: A Formula Approach* available from Blue Poppy Press.

Problem Based Learning Exercises (See App. IV for answers)

1. What are the three major categories of potential toxicity of which practitioners of Chinese medicine need to be aware?
2. Medicinals that are suspected by the FDA to be nephrotoxic contain what substance?
3. Name a specific medicinal which contains this substance

4. If I were planning to use a formula containing *He Zi* or *Di Yu*, what Western medications would I need to make sure that my patient was NOT taking?

A.

B.

C.

D.

E.

5. Known risk factors for hepatotoxic reactions that we need to be aware of in our patients include:

A.

B.

C.

D.

6. The appearance of what signs and symptoms of potential medicine-induced hepatitis tell us that we should stop the use of an herbal formula?

A.

B.

C.

D.

7. Name several specific herbal medicinals that are highly toxic and should not be used during pregnancy.

8. What class of Chinese medicinals are generally not used with patients taking warfarin-based Western pharmaceuticals?

Exercises

1. Go on-line and find out the signs and symptoms of nephrotoxicity and kidney failure.

2. Go on-line and find out everything you can about the Belgium AA incident and other cases of nephrotoxicity attributed to Chinese herbal medicine.

3. What are the clinical signs and symptoms of hepatitis?

4. Search on-line for the compound keywords of "fetotoxicity + Chinese herbal medicine" or "fetotoxicity + Chinese herbs."

A. Is there any information?

B. How valid does that information appear to be?

5. What do you intend to tell your patients about nephro-, hepa-to-, and/or fetotoxicity if they ask?

CHAPTER 9

Chinese Herbal Medicine During Pregnancy & Lactation

Many practitioners and their patients worry about the safety of Chinese herbal medicinals during pregnancy and lactation. These are understandable concerns. However, a lot of misunderstanding has grown up around them.

Prohibited herbs during pregnancy

When we go to school, we learn that certain Chinese medicinals are prohibited during pregnancy and that others are to be used with caution only. Unfortunately, these prohibitions are not as clear-cut and universal as they outwardly seem. Many of these prohibitions are for the "uninitiated," the "outsiders." If we have studied Chinese medical gynecology, a number of these prohibitions are allowed and even necessary when warranted.

In order to understand this, we must understand what the word "warrant" means. In law, a warrant is permission to do something which is otherwise illegal. For instance, if the police have a warrant they can "kidnap" a person, *i.e.*, put them in jail against their will. Or, if police have a warrant, they can "break and enter" to conduct a search. In order to obtain a warrant, one must present evidence that the otherwise prohibited action is necessary or warranted.

Let's take a concrete example from the world of Chinese medicine. *Ban Xia* (Rhizoma Pinelliae Ternatae) is sometimes considered prohibited during pregnancy due to its containing toxins. However, it is the main ingredient for harmonizing the stomach and stopping vomiting. This means that, without nausea and vomiting, one should not use *Ban Xia* during pregnancy, but, *if there is nausea and vomiting, during pregnancy, Ban Xia* becomes a main and necessary ingredient. As an extension of this, as soon as the nausea and vomiting are eliminated, the *Ban Xia* should be discontinued because it is now unwarranted.

Here's another example. *Dan Pi* (Cortex Radicis Moutan) is prohibited during pregnancy due to its quickening of the blood. It is assumed that quickening of the blood may lead to miscarriage. However, in Chinese gynecology, one of the three causes of miscarriage is blood stasis. (The other two are qi vacuity and heat.) Because *Dan Pi* quickens the blood and dispels stasis, clears heat and stops bleeding, its use is warranted during pregnancy *when used to forestall a miscarriage due to heat stasis.* In that case, to avoid using *Dan Pi* because of the textbook prohibition may actually lead to the occurrence of the miscarriage. In other words, the use of *Dan Pi* may not only be warranted but actually necessary, and to avoid its use may lead to exactly the thing we were trying to prevent or avoid. Similarly, *Qu Mai* (Herba Dianthi) and *Che Qian Zi* (Semen Plantaginis) are only prohibited if there is no water swelling and/or strangury, and *Mang Xiao* (Mirabilitum) is only prohibited if there is no constipation due to yang ming heat repletion. If there is water swelling and/or strangury or there is constipation due to yang ming replete heat, then these medicinals are warranted and should be used.

The only Chinese medicinals that are *always and completely prohibited* during pregnancy are those that are so toxic they may potentially kill the fetus, such as *Xiong Huang* (Realgar) and *Tian Hua Fen* (Radix Trichosanthis Kirlowii).

Chinese herbs during breast-feeding

There is no discussion in the Chinese medical literature of which I am aware about Chinese herbs that are prohibited during breast-feeding. Basically, I would say that the test as to whether a Chinese medicinal is OK or not during lactation is the same as above—whether or not it is warranted. According to Chinese medical theory, the milk is made out of the mother's blood. If the mother is ill, she is out of balance, and it is logical that this imbalance may reflect itself in the quality and composition of the mother's milk. Therefore, anything which brings the mother back to balance and harmony should also result in better quality, more healthful milk. Thus, I never hesitate to give a lactating woman a particular Chinese herb if that medicinal is indicated by the combination of both her disease and her personally presenting pattern. After 25 years in practice, I have never seen any problems with this approach.

> **Anything which brings the mother back to balance and harmony should also result in better quality, more healthful milk.**

Case History Exercises (See App. IV for answers)

Case 1: Female, 32 years old

The patient presents with a threatened spontaneous abortion or miscarriage. She is eight weeks pregnant and has had at least one previous miscarriage six months before. There is lower abdominal pain which is fixed in location as well as leakage of pinkish, dilute blood. The patient has a pale, fat tongue with thin, white fur and a fine, forceless, bowstring pulse. The leakage is worse when she stands up and was initiated by overwork. The patient says she is generally fatigued. She has a pale but dusky facial complexion as if she had soot on her face. She says that she has a long history of painful menstruation. Whenever her menses aren't painful, she has bad PMS.

1. What are the three main mechanisms of any and all types of gynecological bleeding?
2. What is this patient's Chinese medical disease diagnosis?
3. What are the patient's patterns associated with her threatened miscarriage?
4. What signs and symptoms indicate what patterns?
5. What are the treatment principles for those patterns?
6. What Chinese medicinal stops bleeding at the same time as it quickens the blood?
7. Do you think you can use this medicinal in this case?
8. If not, what medicinal(s) do you propose?
9. If yes, how long do you propose to use it?

Case 2: Female, 39 years old

The patient is also eight weeks pregnant and has severe "morning sickness." She is nauseous all day long and sometimes desires to vomit. However, when she tries to, all she does is dry heave. Her nausea is worse at night. The patient has a dry mouth and is thirsty, but all she can do is sip. In the past, the woman has had to use steroids for long periods of time because she suffers from relapsing/remittent lupus erythematous. The woman feels a gnawing hunger in her stomach, but cannot eat anything except small bits at a time. In addition, the woman tends to have a flushed facial complexion, dry skin and hair, and dry, brittle nails. Her tongue is dry, red, and almost completely denuded of fur, while her pulse is fine, slippery, and rapid.

1. What is this patient's Chinese medical disease diagnosis?
2. What is/are her presenting pattern(s)?
3. What are the treatment principles for this/these pattern(s)?
4. Which of the two Chinese medicinals will you choose for this woman, *Tian Hua Fen* (Radix Trichosanthis Kirlowii) or *Mai Men Dong* (Tuber Ophiopogonis Japonici), and why?

5. Please write a representative Chinese herbal formula for this woman.

6. Should this woman take her Chinese herbs in powdered extract or decoction form? Why?

7. If you choose to give this woman her Chinese medicinals in decoction, at what dosage and intervals?

8. If she says that the smell of the Chinese medicinals make her nauseous what might you advise?

9. Must this woman take her decocted Chinese herbs warm or not? Why?

Case 3: Female, 27 years old

The patient is a breast-feeding mother with a three-month-old child. She suffers from chronic, recalcitrant psoriasis which has gotten worse during pregnancy and breast-feeding. The woman has had psoriasis ever since she was a teenager. The lesions consist of dry patches of silvery scales surrounded by dark red, angry-looking margins. The woman wants treatment for her condition but is worried about taking Chinese herbs while she is breast-feeding.

1. What are the disease mechanisms associated with this woman's psoriasis?

2. What are the treatment principles?

3. Do you think external application of Chinese medicinals will be adequate to control or eliminate this situation?

4. If not, based on the above treatment principles, are there any medicinals you are worried might harm the baby?

5. Are any of the mother's disease mechanisms associated with this condition transferrable to the child via the milk according to Chinese medical theory? If so, what are they? What are the medicinals typically used in Chinese medicine to treat skin diseases associated with this/these mechanism(s)?

6. Is treatment of the mother for any of her disease mech-

anisms likely to have a salutary effect on the child via the breast milk? If so, which ones and why or how?

7. Is treatment of the mother for any of her disease mechanisms likely to have a deleterious effect on the child via the breast milk? If so, which ones and why or how?

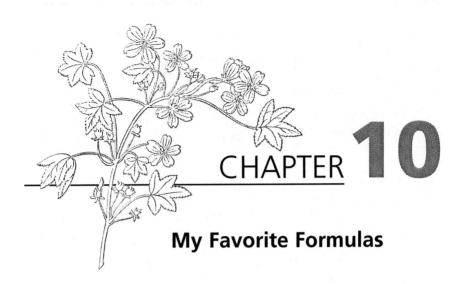

CHAPTER **10**

My Favorite Formulas

It is commonly said that new practitioners use many formulas, but old practitioners only use a few. In my experience, this is very true. The explanation for this is that old practitioners with many years of clinical experience have realized that most patients (at least those with chronic conditions) present only a small group of patterns. In fact, the most commonly presenting pattern in such patients is a wood-earth disharmony. What this means is either a liver-spleen, liver-stomach disharmony, or liver-spleen-stomach disharmony. It is rare to find a middle-aged adult without one of these patterns at the root of their disease mechanisms. This is why it is said that, "In adults, blame the liver," "The liver is the thief of the five viscera and six bowels," and "Depression makes for hundreds of diseases."

> It is commonly said that new practitioners use many formulas, but old practitioners only use a few.

Further, according to the *Ling Shu (Spiritual Pivot)*, "[When] disease first occurs in the liver, in three days, it will also be in the spleen." Along the same vein, Zhang Zhong-jing, in the *Jin Gui Yao Lue (Essentials of the Golden Cabinet)* stated, "[When] liver disease appears, know that the liver transmits

> **Ling Shu (Spiritual Pivot), "[When] disease first occurs in the liver, in three days, it will also be in the spleen."**

to the spleen. [Therefore,] one must first replete the spleen." Thus it is also said, "Liver disease *is* spleen disease." Because of the close relationship between the liver, spleen, and stomach *vis á vis* the qi mechanism, it is rare to have an enduring disease in any of these viscera without disease in the others. The liver governs coursing and discharge which keeps the qi mechanism freely flowing and uninhibited. The spleen governs upbearing, the stomach governs downbearing, and the qi mechanism is nothing other than the upbearing, downbearing, entering, and exiting of the qi. This is why Zhang Xi-chun said,

[If] one desires to treat the liver, one must first upbear the spleen and downbear the stomach, bank and nourish the central palace. When the central palace's qi transformation becomes generous, liver wood is automatically rectified.

When there is a liver-spleen or liver-stomach disharmony, the treatment principle is to either *harmonize* the liver and spleen or *harmonize* the liver and stomach. In terms of clinical practice, that means picking the guiding formula from the harmonizing category of formulas. There are five main types of harmonizing formulas:

1. Defensive & constructive harmonizing formulas
2. Liver & spleen harmonizing formulas
3. Liver & stomach harmonizing formulas
4. Spleen & stomach harmonizing formulas
5. Stomach & intestines harmonizing formulas

In general, it is from these harmonizing formulas that older practitioners typically choose a starting place for the majority of their patients. When we know how to modify the main formulas in the harmonizing category with various additions and subtractions, we can treat 80-85% of our patient load successfully. This is the reason why *Xiao Chai Hu Tang* (Minor Bupleurum Decoction), perhaps the most famous harmonizing formula, is the single most commonly prescribed formula in Chinese medicine as evidenced by Japanese insurance reimbursement records. That being said, what are my favorite formulas?

Xiao Chai Hu Tang (Minor Bupleurum Decoction)

Although this formula was first introduced in the *Shang Han Lun (Treatise on Damage [Due to] Cold)* as the prototypical *shao yang* aspect harmonizing formula, in day to day clinical practice, it is more commonly used to treat a liver-spleen or liver-stomach disharmony complicated with heat in the liver/gallbladder, stomach, lungs, and/or heart. That heat may be either depressive or damp heat. In addition, there may also be the complication of phlegm, dampness, and turbidity. Within this formula:

- *Chai Hu* (Radix Bupleuri) courses the liver and rectifies the qi by upbearing yang and out-thrusting depression.
- *Dang Shen* (Radix Codonopsitis Pilosulae) fortifies the spleen and supplements the qi.
- *Huang Qin* (Radix Scutellariae Baicalensis) clears externally contracted or retained heat evils and depressive or damp heat from the liver/gallbladder, stomach and intestines, lungs, and/or heart.
- *Ban Xia* (Rhizoma Pinelliae Ternatae) harmonizes the stomach and downbears counterflow, transforms phlegm and dispels dampness.
- *Sheng Jiang* (uncooked Rhizoma Zingiberis Officinalis) aids *Ban Xia* in all these activities.
- Mix-fried *Gan Cao* (Radix Glycyrrhizae Uralensis) and *Da Zao* (Fructus Zizyphi Jujubae) aid *Dang Shen* in fortifying the spleen and supplementing the qi. They also supplement the heart and quiet the spirit. Since the heart gets its qi and blood from the clear upborne by the spleen, spleen vacuity is commonly complicated by some element of heart qi vacuity.

Common modifications of *Xiao Chai Hu Tang*

Xiao Chai Hu Tang may be modified in numerous ways. The following are only some of the best known, most common modifications:[1]

1. If **phlegm and/or dampness** are pronounced, add *Fu Ling* (Sclerotium Poriae Cocos) and *Chen Pi* (Pericarpium Citri Reticulatae).

2. If there is **pronounced thirst** due to heat and no phlegm dampness, subtract *Ban Xia* and add *Tian Hua Fen* (Radix Tricho - santhis Kirlowii). If there is thirst and phlegm or dampness, keep *Ban Xia* and add *Mai Men Dong* (Tuber Ophiopogonis Japonici) and/or *Tian Hua Fen* (Radix Trichosanthis Kirlowii).

3. If there is **qi stagnation abdominal cramping pain**, add *Bai Shao* (Radix Albus Paeoniae Lactiflorae).

4. Also for **abdominal pain associated with qi stagnation and dampness**, add *Sha Ren* (Fructus Amomi) and *Mu Xiang* (Radix Auklandiae Lappae).

5. For **abdominal distention and pain** due to qi stagnation, add *Yan Hu Suo* (Rhizoma Corydalis Yanhusuo), *Xiang Fu* (Rhizoma Cyperi Rotundi, and *Zhi Shi* (Fructus Immaturus Citri Aurantii).

6. For **scanty, reddish yellow, astringent, and painful urina- tion**, add *Jin Qian Cao* (Herba Lysimachiae) and *Bai Hua She She Cao* (Herba Oldenlandiae Diffusae Cum Radice).

7. For **constipation with yellow tongue fur**, add either *Da*

---

[1] You will notice that most of the modifications listed for each formula in this chapter are two-herb cobinations. Based on empirical experience these combinations' therapeutic effect is oftn better than either single medicinal on its own. For a detailed discussion of this subject, see *Dui Yao: The Art of Combining Chinese Medicinals* by Philippe Sionneau.

Huang (Radix Et Rhizoma Rhei) or *Huo Ma Ren* (Semen Cannabis Sativae) and *Zhi Shi* (Fructus Immaturus Citri Aurantii).

8. For **fever, cough with yellow phlegm, and pain in the chest**, add *Jie Geng* (Radix Platycodi Grandiflori), *Gua Lou* (Fructus Trichosanthis Kirlowii), and *Zhe Bei Mu* (Bulbus Fritillariae Thunbergii).

9. For **malaria-like diseases**,[2] add *Qing Hao* (Herba Artemisiae Apiacae) and *Chang Shan* (Radix Dichroae Febrifugae).

10. Also for **malaria-like diseases**, add *Chang Shan* (Radix Dichroae Febrifugae) and *Cao Guo* (Fructus Amomi Tsaokuo).

11. For **malaria-like diseases with a heavy sensation in the limbs, loss of appetite, and a soggy pulse**, subtract *Sheng Jiang* and *Da Zao* and add *Cang Zhu* (Rhizoma Atractylodis) and *Hou Po* (Cortex Magnoliae Officinalis). This results in *Chai Ping Tang* (Bupleurum Leveling Decoction).

12. For **dizziness and vertigo**, add *Ju Hua* (Flos Chrysanthemi Morifolii), *Gou Teng* (Ramulus Uncariae Seu Uncis), and *Jue Ming Zi* (Semen Cassiae Torae).

13. For concomitant **yin vacuity**, add *Bie Jia* (Carapax Amydae Sinensis) and *Qing Hao* (Herba Artemisiae Annuae Seu Apiacae).

14. For **chest oppression and stomach duct fullness**, add *Xiang Fu* (Rhizoma Cyperi Rotundi) and *Zhi Shi* (Fructus Immaturus Citri Aurantii).

15. For concomitant **kidney yang vacuity with cockcrow diarrhea**, lower abdominal bloating, and thirst, add *Fu Ling* (Sclerotium Poriae Cocos), *Ze Xie* (Rhizoma Alismatis Orientalis),

---

2 Definition of malaria-like diseases: Malaria-like diseases include any disease in which there is remittent, relapsing fevers and possibly chills which occur on a regular basis.

Shan Yao (Radix Dioscoreae Oppositae), and *Tu Si Zi* (Semen Cuscutae Chinensis).

16. For **lung qi and defensive exterior vacuity**, add *Wu Wei Zi* (Fructus Schisandrae Chinensis) and *Huang Qi* (Radix Astragali Membranacei).

17. For **severe fatigue**, add *Huang Qi* (Radix Astragali Membranacei).

18. For **recurrent lung heat diseases**, add *Huang Lian* (Rhizoma Coptidis Chinensis) and *Gua Lou Ren* (Semen Trichosanthis Kirlowii). This results in *Chai Xian Tang* (Bupleurum Fall Decoction).

19. For **cough with sticky, hard-to-expectorate phlegm**, add *Gua Lou Ren* (Semen Trichosanthis Kirlowii), *Jie Geng* (Radix Platycodi Grandiflori), and *Zhi Shi* (Fructus Immaturus Citri Aurantii).

20. For **dry cough**, add *Mai Men Dong* (Tuber Ophiopogonis Japonici) and *Zhu Ru* (Caulis Bambusae In Taeniis).

21. For **sinusitis with a yellow nasal discharge** due to gallbladder heat invading the brain,[3] add *Cang Er Zi* (Fructus Xanthii Sibirici) and *Bo He* (Herba Menthae Haplocalycis).

22. For **muscle tension and chronic intestinal disorders** with chilled extremities, add *Gui Zhi* (Ramulus Cinnamomi Cassiae) and *Bai Shao* (Radix Albus Paeoniae Lactiflorae). This results in *Chai Hu Gui Zhi Tang* (Bupleurum & Cinnamon Decoction).

---

[3] Definition of gallbladder heat invading the brain: Gallbladder heat invading the brain refers to sinusitis. In early China, doctors did not understand the function of the brain, and, to them, it looked like a large repository of phlegm. Therefore, nasal discharge was called fetal leakage. When depressive heat from the liver flows the gallbladder channel upward to steam and brew in the cavities of the head, *i.e.*, the sinuses, this cooks the phlegm and turns it yellow, green, and purulent.

23. For **pleurisy and wilting diseases**[4] **involving the lungs**, add *Qin Jiao* (Radix Gentianae Qinjiao), *Di Gu Pi* (Cortex Radicis Lycii Chinensis), *Zi Wan* (Radix Asteris Tartarici), *Bie Jia* (Carapax Amydae Sinensis), *Dang Gui* (Radix Angelicae Sinensis), and *Wu Mei* (Fructus Pruni Mume). This results in *Qin Jiao Fu Lei Tang* (Gentiana Macrophylla Support Marked Emaciation Decoction).

24. If there is **dry-stool constipation**, add *Mang Xiao* (Mirabilitum). This results in *Chai Hu Jia Mang Xiao Tang* (Bupleurum & Mirabilitum Decoction).

25. If there is **alternating fever and chills, headache in the lateral sides of the forehead, vertigo,** fullness and pain in the chest and rib-side regions, white tongue fur, and a bowstring, slippery pulse on the right and a bowstring, floating, large pulse on the left, subtract *Ren Shen* and *Da Zao* and add *Zhi Ke* (Fructus Citri Aurantii), *Jie Geng* (Radix Platycodi Grandiflori), and *Chen Pi* (Pericarpium Citri Reticulatae). This results in *Chai Hu Zhi Jie Tang* (Bupleurum, Citrus & Platycodon Decoction).

26. If a **female patient catches a cold before or with each period** accompanied by alternating fever and chills, lack of appetite, and a bowstring pulse, add the ingredients of *Si Wu Tang* (Four Materials Decoction), *i.e.*, *Dang Gui* (Radix Angelicae Sinensis), *Bai Shao* (Radix Albus Paeoniae Lactiflorae), *Shu Di* (cooked Radix Rehmanniae Glutinosae), and *Chuan Xiong* (Radix Ligustici Wallichii).

27. For **constipation or diarrhea which burns the anus**, abdominal glomus and fullness which feels hard to the touch, nausea, continuous vomiting, a bitter taste in the mouth,

---

[4] Definition of wilting diseases: Wilting diseases are those accompanied by muscular wasting and atrophy which lead to loss of function, including movement and sensation. Lung diseases typically involve heat, and enduring heat consumes and damages yin, blood, and fluids. If such a yin-blood vacuity fails to nourish and moisten the muscles and sinews, these may become wilted and atrophied.

despondency and slight irritability, yellow tongue fur, and a bowstring, forceful pulse, subtract *Ren Shen* and add *Da Huang* (Radix Et Rhizoma Rhei), *Bai Shao* (Radix Albus Paeoniae Lactiflorae), and *Zhi Shi* (Fructus Immaturus Citri Aurantii). This results in *Da Chai Hu Tang* (Major Bupleurum Decoction).

28. If there is **severe vomiting and constipation**, to *Da Chai Hu Tang* add *Huang Lian* (Rhizoma Coptidis Chinensis) and *Wu Zhu Yu* (Fructus Evodiae Rutecarpae).

29. If there is **severe pain and constipation**, to *Da Chai Hu Tang* add *Dang Gui* (Radix Angelicae Sinensis) and *Yan Hu Suo* (Rhizoma Corydalis Yanhusuo) or *Chi Shao* (Radix Rubrus Paeoniae Lactiflorae) and *Tao Ren* (Semen Pruni Persicae).

30. For **menstrual irregularity and premenstrual tension**, add *Xiang Fu* (Rhizoma Cyperi Rotundi) and *Bai Shao* (Radix Albus Paeoniae Lactiflorae) or *Bai Shao* and *Dang Gui* (Radix Angelicae Sinensis).

31. For **premenstrual breast distention**, add *Chuan Lian Zi* (Fructus Meliae Toosendan) and *Xia Ku Cao* (Spica Prunellae Vulgaris).

32. For **vexatious heat before menstruation**, reduce the dosages of *Ban Xia* and *Ren Shen* and add *Dan Pi* (Cortex Radicis Moutan), *Zhi Zi* (Fructus Gardeniae Jasminoidis), and *Sheng Di* (uncooked Radix Rehmanniae Glutinosae).

33. For **edema**, add *Fu Ling* (Sclerotium Poriae Cocos) and *Ze Xie* (Rhizoma Alismatis Orientalis).

34. For **heart palpitations and insomnia**, add *Yuan Zhi* (Radix Polygalae Tenuifoliae), *Suan Zao Ren* (Semen Zizyphi Spinosae), and *Dang Gui* (Radix Angelicae Sinensis).

35. For **premenstrual mental dullness and headache**, add *Ju*

Hua (Flos Chrysanthemi Morifolii) and *Chuan Xiong* (Radix Ligustici Wallichii).

36. For **clots in the menstruate**, add *Dan Shen* (Radix Salviae Miltiorrhizae) and *Ji Xue Teng* (Caulis Millettiae Seu Spatholobi) or *Pu Huang* (Pollen Typhae) and *Wu Ling Zhi* (Feces Trogopterori Seu Pteromi).

37. For **infertility due to liver-spleen disharmony plus kidney yin and yang vacuity**, add *Zi Shi Ying* (Fluoritum) and *Nu Zhen Zi* (Fructus Ligustri Lucidi).

These modifications are only meant to give some idea of the modifiability of this formula and are not comprehensive.

Xiao Yao San (Rambling Powder)

This harmonizing formula harmonizes the liver and spleen and the qi and blood. Harmonizing the qi and blood in this case means rectifying the qi and nourishing the blood. This formula is indicated for patients exhibiting a liver-spleen disharmony complicated by blood vacuity and dampness.

Within this formula:
• *Chai Hu* (Radix Bupleuri) courses the liver and rectifies the qi.
• *Dang Gui* (Radix Angelicae Sinensis) and *Bai Shao* (Radix Albus Paeoniae Lactiflorae) supplement the blood and nourish the liver.
• *Bai Zhu* (Rhizoma Atractylodis Macrocephalae), *Fu Ling* (Sclerotium Poriae Cocos), mix-fried *Gan Cao* (Radix Glycyrrhizae Uralensis), and *Sheng Jiang* (uncooked Rhizoma Zingiberis Officinalis) fortify the spleen, supplement the qi, and dispel dampness by both seeping and transforming it.
• *Bo He* (Herba Menthae Haplocalycis) aids *Chai Hu* in coursing and draining the liver qi.

Common modifications of *Xiao Yao San*

The following are some of this formula's well known modifications:

1. If there is **depressive heat**, especially if this heat enters the blood aspect, add *Zhi Zi* (Fructus Gardeniae Jasminoidis) and *Dan Pi* (Cortex Radicis Moutan). This results in *Dan Zhi Xiao Yao San* (Moutan & Gardenia Rambling Powder).

2. If there is more **serious blood vacuity**, add *Shu Di* (cooked Radix Rehmanniae Glutinosae). This results in *Hei Xiao Yao San* (Black Rambling Powder).

3. For concomitant **qi vacuity**, add *Ren Shen* (Radix Panacis Ginseng) or *Dang Shen* (Radix Codonopsitis Pilosulae) and/or *Huang Qi* (Radix Astragali Membranacei).

4. Also for **qi vacuity**, add *Dang Shen* (Radix Codonopsitis Pilosulae) and *Tai Zi Shen* (Radix Pseudostellariae).

5. For **qi vacuity and spleen weakness with borborygmus and loose stools**, subtract *Bo He* and add *Huang Qi* (Radix Astragali Membranacei) and *Sheng Ma* (Rhizoma Cimicifugae).

6. For **rib-side pain**, add *Yan Hu Suo* (Rhizoma Corydalis Yanhusuo) and *Chuan Lian Zi* (Fructus Meliae Toosendan).

7. For **intense, fixed pain due to blood stasis**, add *Dan Pi* (Cortex Radicis Moutan), *Yu Jin* (Tuber Curcumae), and *San Leng* (Rhizoma Sparganii Stoloniferi).

8. For **cold mounting pain due to cold and dampness attacking the small intestine**, subtract *Bai Shao, Bo He*, and *Chai Hu* and add *Chuan Lian Zi* (Fructus Meliae Toosendan), *Wu Zhu Yu* (Fructus Evodiae Rutecarpae), *Mu Xiang* (Radix Auklandiae Lappae), and *Xiao Hui Xiang* (Fructus Foeniculi Vulgaris).

9. For **abnormal vaginal discharge**, add *Jin Yin Hua* (Flos Lonicerae Japonicae) and *Guan Zhong* (Rhizoma Guanchong).

10. Also for **abnormal vaginal discharge**, add *Bi Xie* (Rhizoma Dioscoreae Hypoglaucae), *Che Qian Zi* (Semen Plantaginis), and *Chun Pi* (Cortex Cedrelae).

11. If abnormal **vaginal discharge is due to downward perco-lation of spleen-kidney vacuity** and concomitant damp heat, add *Shan Yao* (Radix Dioscoreae Oppositae), *Qian Shi* (Semen Euryalis Ferocis), and *Che Qian Zi* (Semen Plantaginis).

12. For **vaginal itching and burning urination**, add *Long Dan Cao* (Radix Gentianae Scabrae), *Zhi Zi* (Fructus Gardeniae Jasminoidis), *Huang Qin* (Radix Scutellariae Baicalensis), *Ze Xie* (Rhizoma Alismatis Orientalis), and *Mu Tong* (Caulis Akebiae).

13. For **pain in the area of the liver with reduced appetite and fatigue** as in non-icteric hepatitis, subtract *Sheng Jiang* and *Bo He* and add *Xiang Fu* (Rhizoma Cyperi Rotundi), *Fo Shou* (Fructus Citri Sacrodactylis), *Dan Shen* (Radix Salviae Miltiorrhizae), and *Dang Shen* (Radix Codonopsitis Pilosulae).

14. For an **enlarged liver and spleen**, add *Wu Zei Gu* (Os Sepiae Seu Sepiellae), *Bie Jia* (Carapax Amydae Sinensis), and *Mu Li* (Concha Ostreae).

15. For an **enlarged, hard liver with a dull, black facial com-plexion and cyanotic lips**, add *San Leng* (Rhizoma Sparganii Stoloniferi), *E Zhu* (Rhizoma Curcumae Zedoariae), *Hong Hua* (Flos Carthami Tinctorii), and *Dan Shen* (Radix Salviae Miltiorrhizae).

16. For **fibrocystic breasts** due to qi stagnation and blood stasis, subtract *Gan Cao* and add *Wang Bu Liu Xing* (Semen Vaccariae Segetalis), *Ji Xue Teng* (Caulis Millettiae Seu Spatholobi), *Dan Shen* (Radix Salviae Miltiorrhizae), and *Xiang Fu* (Rhizoma Cyperi Rotundi).

17. For **premenstrual breast distention and pain**, add *Gua Lou* (Fructus Trichosanthis Kirlowii) and *Qiang Huo* (Radix Et Rhizoma Notopterygii).

18. For **hypertension**, add *Xia Ku Cao* (Spica Prunellae Vulgaris), *Sang Ji Sheng* (Ramulus Loranthi Seu Visci), and *Nu Zhen Zi* (Fructus Ligustri Lucidi).

19. For various **ophthalmological disorders**, such as glaucoma, optic nerve atrophy, acute retrobulbar neuritis, cortical blindness, and central retinitis, add *Ju Hua* (Flos Chrysanthemi Morifolii), *Gou Qi Zi* (Fructus Lycii Chinensis), and *Shi Chang Pu* (Rhizoma Acori Graminei).

20. For **red eyes and mental dullness due to upward rising of depressive heat** of the heart, liver, and spleen, add *Chuan Xiong* (Radix Ligustici Wallichii), *Ju Hua* (Flos Chrysanthemi Morifolii), *Jin Yin Hua* (Flos Lonicerae Japonicae), *Huang Qin* (Radix Scutellariae Baicalensis), and *Huang Lian* (Rhizoma Coptidis Chinensis).

21. For **insomnia**, add *Mu Li* (Concha Ostreae) and *Long Gu* (Os Draconis).

22. For **insomnia and profuse dreams**, add *Suan Zao Ren* (Semen Zizyphi Spinosae) and *Bai Zi Ren* (Semen Biotae Orientalis).

23. For **insomnia, profuse dreams, mental dullness, and dizziness**, add *Suan Zao Ren Tang* (Zizyphus Spinosa Decoction), *i.e.*, *Suan Zao Ren* (Semen Zizyphi Spinosae), *Chuan Xiong* (Radix Ligustici Wallichii), and *Zhi Mu* (Rhizoma Anemarrhena Aspheloidis).

24. For **abdominal distention**, add *Hou Po* (Cortex Magnoliae Officinalis) and *Chen Pi* (Pericarpium Citri Reticulatae).

25. For **abdominal distention and decreased food intake**, add *Ban Xia* (Rhizoma Pinelliae Ternatae), *Bai Dou Kou* (Fructus Cardamomi), and *Mai Ya* (Fructus Germinatus Hordei Vulgaris).

26. For **abdominal distention, fatigue, and decreased food intake**, add *Dang Shen* (Radix Codonopsitis Pilosulae), *Mai Ya* (Fructus Germinatus Hordei Vulgaris), and *Ji Nei Jin* (Endothelium Corneum Gigeriae Galli).

27. For **abdominal distention, loose stools, borborygmus, and flatulence**, add *Xiang Sha Liu Jun Zi Tang* (Auklandia & Amomum Six Gentlemen Decoction), *i.e.*, *Ren Shen* (Radix Panacis Ginseng), *Ban Xia* (Rhizoma Pinelliae Ternatae), *Chen Pi* (Pericarpium Citri Reticulatae), *Sha Ren* (Fructus Amomi), and *Mu Xiang* (Radix Auklandiae Lappae).

28. For **acne** due to depressive heat steaming the lungs, use *Dan Zhi Xiao Yao San* and add *Niu Bang Zi* (Fructus Arctii Lappae) and *Lian Qiao* (Fructus Forsythiae Suspensae).

29. For **diarrhea** due to spleen vacuity and dampness, add *Ban Xia* (Rhizoma Pinelliae Ternatae) and *Shan Yao* (Radix Dioscoreae Oppositae) or *Shan Yao* and *Bai Bian Dou* (Semen Dolichoris Lablab).

30. If there is **headache accompanying menstruation**, add *Jing Jie Sui* (Herba Seu Flos Schizonepetae Tenuifoliae) and *Bai Zhi* (Radix Angelicae Dahuricae).

31. If there is **nervous excitability**, add *Chuan Xiong* (Radix Ligustici Wallichii) and *Gou Teng* (Ramulus Uncariae Cum Uncis).

32. For **nervous anxiety and agitation** due to liver qi disturbing the heart spirit, add *Hu Po* (Succinum) and *Yuan Zhi* (Radix Polygalae Tenuifoliae).

33. For **yin vacuity** with a red tongue and scanty fur, add *Nu Zhen*

Zi (Fructus Ligustri Lucidi), *Han Lian Cao* (Herba Ecliptae Prostratae), and *Gou Qi Zi* (Fructus Lycii Chinensis).

34. For **edema of the lower extremities and scanty urination**, add *Qu Mai* (Herba Dianthi), *Bian Xu* (Herba Polygoni Avicularis), *Ze Xie* (Rhizoma Alismatis Orientalis), and *Che Qian Zi* (Semen Plantaginis).

35. For **nose-bleeding and bleeding gums** due to liver-stomach depressive heat, add *Sheng Di* (uncooked Radix Rehmanniae Glutinosae), *Dan Pi* (Cortex Radicis Moutan), and *Bai Mao Gen* (Rhizoma Imperatae Cylindricae).

36. If there is **nose-bleeding** due to depressive heat of the heart, lung, and liver, add *Qian Cao Gen* (Radix Rubiae Cordifoliae).

37. For **premenstrual nose-bleeding**, add carbonized *Zhi Zi* (Fructus Gardeniae Jasminoidis), *Bai Mao Gen* (Rhizoma Imperatae Cylindricae), *Xiao Ji* (Herba Cephalanoplos Segeti), and *Chuan Niu Xi* (Radix Cyathulae).

38. For **dry mouth and thirst** due to stomach fluid dryness, add *Sheng Di* (uncooked Radix Rehmanniae Glutinosae) and *Tian Hua Fen* (Radix Trichosanthis Kirlowii).

39. For **headache and vertigo**, add *Tian Ma* (Rhizoma Gastrodiae Elatae), *Gou Teng* (Ramulus Uncariae Cum Uncis), and *Ju Hua* (Flos Chrysanthemi Morifolii).

40. If there is a **flushed face, heart vexation, and easy anger** due to heat evils harassing the heart spirit, add *Huang Lian* (Rhizoma Coptidis Chinensis) and *Long Dan Cao* (Radix Gentianae Scabrae) to *Dan Zhi Xiao Yao San*.

41. For internal confinement of **damp heat with jaundice**, add *Huang Bai* (Cortex Phellodendri), *Yin Chen Hao* (Herba Artemisiae Capillaris), and *Zhi Zi* (Fructus Gardeniae Jasminoidis).

42. For flooding (*i.e.*, **uterine bleeding**) due to anger damaging
the liver or **continuous, purple-colored spotting with clots**,
lower abdominal distention, chest and stomach duct fullness
and oppression, shortness of breath, decreased food intake,
fatigue, and indigestion, subtract *Dang Gui* and *Gan Cao* and add
Nan Sha Shen (Radix Adenophorae Strictae), stir-fried *Pu Huang*
(Pollen Typhae), *Xue Yu Tan* (Crinis Carbonisatus), and black-
ened *Ai Ye* (Folium Artemisiae Argyii). This results in *Fu Pi Shu
Gan Tang* (Support the Spleen & Soothe the Liver Decoction).

43. For **continuous bleeding and spotting** due to depressive
heat entering the blood aspect with distention and pain in the
lower abdomen, add *Huang Qin* (Radix Scutellariae Baicalensis)
and *Huang Bai* (Cortex Phellodendri).

44. For **bleeding during pregnancy** due to depressive heat and
blood stasis, subtract *Dang Gui* and *Gan Cao* and add *Zhi Zi*
(Fructus Gardeniae Jasminoidis) and *Yi Mu Cao* (Herba Leonuri
Heterophylli). This results in *Shu Yu Qing Gan Yin* (Soothe
Depression & Clear the Liver Drink).

45. For **hot strangury**, add *Che Qian Zi* (Semen Plantaginis) to
Dan Zhi Xiao Yao San.

46. For **early, late, or erratic menstruation with distention
and pain** and the sensation of heat in the lower abdomen, add
Xiang Fu (Rhizoma Cyperi Rotundi), *Yu Jin* (Tuber Curcumae),
and *Jing Jie Sui* (Herba Seu Flos Schizonepetae Tenuifoliae).

47. For **early menstruation with a heavy, red discharge**, add
Sheng Di (uncooked Radix Rehmanniae Glutinosae) and *Bie Jia*
(Carapax Amydae Sinensis).

48. For **scanty menstruation with purplish clots and abdominal pain**, add *Chuan Xiong* (Radix Ligustici Wallichii) and *Yu Jin*
(Tuber Curcumae).

49. For **perimenstrual numbness of the extremities** with yang

vacuity and weak qi, add *Gui Zhi* (Ramulus Cinnamomi Cassiae) and *Ju Hong* (Exocarpium Citri Rubri).

50. For **perimenstrual edema** due to earth not engendering metal with non-diffusion of lung qi, add *Rou Gui* (Cortex Cinnamomi Cassiae) and *Bei Sha Shen* (Radix Glehniae Littoralis).

51. For **women with liver depression qi stagnation and cough and vomiting** due to phlegm dampness attacking the lungs and stomach, add *Ju Hong* (Exocarpium Citri Rubri), *Zhe Bei Mu* (Bulbus Fritillariae Thunbergii), and *Ban Xia* (Rhizoma Pinelliae Ternatae).

52. For **women with constipation due to heat in the stomach and intestines,** add *Da Huang* (Radix Et Rhizoma Rhei) and *Mang Xiao* (Mirabilitum).

53. For **galactorrhea**, add a large dose of stir-fried *Mai Ya* (Fructus Germinatus Hordei Vulgaris).

Ban Xia Xie Xin Tang (Pinellia Drain the Heart Decoction)

This formula harmonizes the spleen, stomach, and intestines. That means it treats a spleen qi vacuity weakness complicated by damp heat in the stomach and intestines. Within this formula:

• *Dang Shen* (Radix Codonopsitis Pilosulae) or *Ren Shen* (Radix Panacis Giseng) and mix-fried *Gan Cao* (Radix Glycyrrhizae Uralensis) fortify the spleen and supplement the qi.

• *Gan Jiang* (dry Rhizoma Zingiberis Officinalis) warms the spleen and helps the foregoing supplementing medicinals achieve their effect. It also moderates the cold and clearing effects of some of the other ingredients in this formula.

• Mix-fried *Gan Cao* and *Da Zao* (Fructus Zizyphi Jujubae) supplement the heart based on the same principle as described above under *Xiao Chai Hu Tang.*

• *Huang Lian* (Rhizoma Coptidis Chinensis) and *Huang Qin*

(Radix Scutellariae Baicalensis) clear heat from the heart and lungs and clear heat and eliminate dampness from stomach and intesines.
• *Ban Xia* (Rhizoma Pinelliae Ternatae) harmonizes the stomach and downbears counterflow.
Therefore, taken as a whole, this formula warms and supplements the spleen at the same time as it clears and drains the stomach and intestines.

Common modifications of *Ban Xia Xie Xin Tang*

Some of the most common modifications of this formula include:

1. For **damp heat accumulating in the middle burner with vomiting**, glomus, and fullness, subtract *Ren Shen* or *Dang Shen, Gan Jiang, Da Zao,* and mix-fried *Gan Cao* and add *Zhi Shi* (Fructus Immaturus Citri Aurantii) and *Sheng Jiang* (uncooked Rhizoma Zingiberis).

2. For more **serious spleen qi vacuity with undigested food in the stool** and irritability, increase the dosage of mix-fried *Gan Cao* to 12-15g. This results in *Gan Cao Xie Xin Tang* (Licorice Drain the Heart Decoction).

3. For water and heat struggling in the middle burner or for **stomach vacuity with food stagnation**, replace *Gan Jiang* with *Sheng Jiang* (uncooked Rhizoma Zingiberis). This results in *Sheng Jiang Xie Xin Tang* (Fresh Ginger Drain the Heart Decoction).

4. For heat in the chest and cold in the stomach with **chest oppression and irritability, nausea, abdominal pain,** white, slimy tongue fur, and a bowstring pulse, subtract *Huang Qin* and add *Gui Zhi* (Ramulus Cinnamomi Cassiae). This results in *Huang Lian Tang* (Coptis Decoction).

5. For **abdominal pain**, add *Sha Ren* (Fructus Amomi) and *Mu Xiang* (Radix Auklandiae Lappae).

6. For **chronic diarrhea**, add *Ge Gen* (Radix Puerariae).

7. For **plum pit qi** and depressive heat, add *Hou Po* (Cortex Magnoliae Officinalis).

8. For a **liver-spleen disharmony with damp heat in the stomach and intestines**, add *Chai Hu* (Radix Bupleuri).

9. For **chest oppression and distention** due to liver depression qi stagnation, add *Chai Hu* and *Gua Lou Ren* (Semen Trichosanthis Kirlowii). This results in *Chai Xian Tang* (Bupleurum Fall Decoction).

Bu Zhong Yi Qi Tang
(Supplement the Center & Boost the Qi Decoction)

This formula is not categorized as a harmonizing formula. Nevertheless, it can be used as one. It is one of the most famous spleen-fortifying, qi-boosting formulas in Chinese medicine. But, because it contains *Chai Hu* (Radix Bupleuri), *Dang Gui* (Radix Angelicae Sinensis), and *Chen Pi* (Pericarpium Citri Reticulatae), this formula also does harmonize the liver and rectify the qi, and any formula which supplements the spleen at the same time as it courses and harmonizes the liver functions as a harmonizing formula whether or not it is categorized as one.

Within this formula:
• *Huang Qi* (Radix Astragali Membranacei), *Ren Shen* (Radix Panacis Ginseng) or *Dang Shen* (Radix Codonopsitis Pilosulae), *Bai Zhu* (Rhizoma Atractylodis Macrocephalae), and mix-fried *Gan Cao* (Radix Glycyrrhizae Uralensis) fortify the spleen and boost the qi.
• *Chai Hu, Chen Pi,* and *Sheng Ma* (Rhizoma Cimicifugae) course the liver and rectify the qi, upbear yang and out-thrust depression.
• *Dang Gui* nourishes the blood and emolliates the liver. When combined with *Chai Hu*, these two medicinals har-

monize the liver, meaning that they harmonize the qi and blood within the liver. In particular, if one wants to course the liver more strongly, all one has to do is raise the dose of *Chai Hu* from 3-4.5 grams to nine grams or more.

Common modifications of *Bu Zhong Yi Qi Tang*

The following are some of the most useful modifications of this formula:

1. If **blood vacuity is prominent**, increase the dosage of *Dang Gui* (Radix Angelicae Sinensis) and add *Bai Shao* (Radix Albus Paeoniae Lactiflorae).

2. For **prolapse** in general, increase the dosage of *Huang Qi* (Radix Astragali Membranacei) and add *Zhi Shi* (Fructus Immaturus Citri Aurantii).

3. For **uterine prolapse**, add *Yi Zhi Ren* (Fructus Alpiniae Oxyphyllae), *Ai Ye* (Folium Artemisiae Argyii), and *Wu Wei Zi* (Fructus Schisandrae Chinensis).

4. For **headache with vertigo and dizziness**, add *Chuan Xiong* (Radix Ligustici Wallichii) and *Ban Xia* (Rhizoma Pinelliae Ternatae).

5. For **vertigo and vomiting**, add *Ge Gen* (Radix Puerariae) and *Ze Xie* (Rhizoma Alismatis Orientalis).

6. For **bodily heaviness, joint pain, irritability, loss of appetite, chest oppression, shortness of the breath**, etc. due to qi stagnation and damp accumulation, replace *Bai Zhu* (Rhizoma Atractylodis Macrocephalae) with *Cang Zhu* (Rhizoma Atractylodis), subtract *Dang Gui* (Radix Angelicae Sinensis), and add *Bai Shao* (Radix Albus Paeoniae Lactiflorae). This results in *Tiao Zhong Yi Qi Tang* (Regulate the Center & Boost the Qi Decoction), another of Li's famous formulas.

7. For **myasthenia gravis**, increase the dosages of *Huang Qi* (Radix Astragali Membranacei) and *Sheng Ma* (Rhizoma Cimicifugae).

8. For **diarrhea** due to excessive thinking and worry resulting in liver-spleen disharmony, add *Mu Xiang* (Radix Auklandiae Lappae).

9. For **diarrhea due to dampness**, subtract *Dang Gui* and add *Fu Ling* (Sclerotium Poriae Cocos), *Cang Zhu* (Rhizoma Atractylodis), and *Yi Zhi Ren* (Fructus Alpiniae Oxyphyllae).

10. For **Prolonged diarrhea with intestinal qi loss of securing and astringency**, add *He Zi* (Fructus Terminaliae Chebulae), *Rou Dou Kou* (Semen Myristicae Fragrantis), *Wu Wei Zi* (Fructus Schisandrae Chinensis), and *Wu Mei* (Fructus Pruni Mume).

11. For **dysentery with tenesmus**, subtract *Dang Gui* and add *Mu Xiang* (Radix Auklandiae Lappae).

12. For **dysentery after the blood and pus have resolved** but there is still foamy mucus, add *Pao Jiang* (blast-fried Rhizoma Zingiberis Officinalis) and *Chi Shi Zhi* (Hallyositum Rubrum).

13. **After dysentery when there is still tenesmus** and mucus in the stools but constipation, add *Fang Feng* (Radix Ledebouriellae Divaricatae).

14. For **cold stomach with qi stagnation**, add *Qing Pi* (Pericarpium Citri Reticulatae Viride), *Sha Ren* (Fructus Amomi), *Mu Xiang* (Radix Auklandiae Lappae), and *Yi Zhi Ren* (Fructus Alpiniae Oxyphyllae).

15. For **ringing in the ears or loss of hearing** due to spleen-kidney qi vacuity, add *Shan Zhu Yu* (Fructus Corni Officinalis) and *Yi Zhi Ren* (Fructus Alpiniae Oxyphyllae).

16. For **diminished eyesight or blurred vision** due to spleen qi and liver blood vacuity, add *Gou Qi Zi* (Fructus Lycii Chinensis) and *Chuan Xiong* (Radix Ligustici Wallichii).

17. For **habitual miscarriage** due to spleen-kidney dual vacuity, add *Du Zhong* (Cortex Eucommiae Ulmoidis) and *Tu Si Zi* (Semen Cuscutae Chinensis).

18. For **restless fetus and threatened abortion**, add *E Jiao* (Gelatinum Corii Asini) and *Ai Ye* (Folium Artemisiae Argyii). This modification can then be made even stronger by adding *Xu Duan* (Radix Dipsaci) and *Sang Ji Sheng* (Ramulus Loranthi Seu Visci).

19. For **abnormal vaginal discharge**, add *Er Miao San* (Two Wonders Powder), *i.e.*, *Cang Zhu* (Rhizoma Atractylodis) and *Huang Bai* (Cortex Phellodendri).

20. For **abdominal distention**, add *Zhi Shi* (Fructus Immaturus Citri Aurantii), *Hou Po* (Cortex Magnoliae Officinalis), *Mu Xiang* (Radix Auklandiae Lappae), and *Sha Ren* (Fructus Amomi).

21. For **mounting disorders**, add *Ju He* (Semen Citri Reticulatae), *Xiao Hui Xiang* (Fructus Foeniculi Vulgaris), and *Li Zhi He* (Semen Litchi Chinensis).

22. For **constipation due to heat** in the yang ming, add processed *Da Huang* (Radix Et Rhizoma Rhei).

23. For **constipation due to spleen vacuity**, add honey and sesame oil.

24. For **painful urinary strangury in the elderly** due to fallen yang qi, add *Ze Xie* (Rhizoma Alismatis Orientalis) and *Mu Tong* (Caulis Akebiae).

25. For **taxation strangury with heat**, add *Zhi Bai Di Huang*

Wan (Anemarrhena & Phellodendron Rehmannia Pills), *i.e., Zhi Mu* (Rhizoma Anemarrhenae Aspheloidis), *Huang Bai* (Cortex Phellodendri), *Shu Di* (cooked Radix Rehmanniae Glutinosae), *Shan Yao* (Radix Dioscoreae Oppositae), *Shan Zhu Yu* (Fructus Corni Officinalis), *Fu Ling* (Sclerotium Poriae Cocos), *Ze Xie* (Rhizoma Alismatis Orientalis), and *Dan Pi* (Cortex Radicis Moutan).

26. For **taxation strangury without heat**, add *Liu Wei Di Huang Wan* (Six Flavors Rehmannia Pills), *i.e., Shu Di* (cooked Radix Rehmanniae Glutinosae), *Shan Yao* (Radix Dioscoreae Oppositae), *Shan Zhu Yu* (Fructus Corni Officinalis), *Fu Ling* (Sclerotium Poriae Cocos), *Ze Xie* (Rhizoma Alismatis Orientalis), and *Dan Pi* (Cortex Radicis Moutan), plus *Mai Men Dong* (Tuber Ophiopogonis Japonici) and *Wu Wei Zi* (Fructus Schisandrae Chinensis).

27. For **frequent urination aggravated by exertion**, add *Shan Yao* (Radix Dioscoreae Oppositae) and *Wu Wei Zi* (Fructus Schisandrae Chinensis).

28. For **dark yellow, concentrated urination after diarrhea** due to damaged fluids, add *Mai Men Dong* (Tuber Ophiopogonis Japonici) and *Wu Wei Zi* (Fructus Schisandrae Chinensis).

29. For **premenstrual diarrhea** when there is a combination of spleen vacuity and stomach and intestinal heat, add *Pao Jiang* (blast-fried Rhizoma Zingiberis Officinalis) and *Huang Lian* (Rhizoma Coptidis Chinensis).

30. For **pediatric bed-wetting**, add *Sang Piao Xiao* (Ootheca Mantidis) and *Yi Zhi Ren* (Fructus Alpiniae Oxyphyllae).

31. For **chronic rhinitis**, add *Cang Er Zi* (Fructus Xanthii Sibirici) and *Xin Yi Hua* (Flos Magnoliae).

32. For **corneal ulcers**, add *Gu Jing Cao* (Scapus Et Inflorescentia

Eriocaulonis Buergeriani), *Jue Ming Zi* (Semen Cassiae Torae), and
Shan Yao (Radix Dioscoreae Oppositae).

33. If there is concomitant **yin vacuity**, either subtract *Chai Hu*
(Radix Bupleuri) and *Sheng Ma* (Rhizoma
Cimicifugae) or reduce their dosages and add *Zhi Mu* (Rhizoma
Anemarrhenae Aspheloidis) and *Huang Bai* (Cortex
Phellodendri).

34. Also for **yin vacuity**, subtract *Chai Hu* and *Sheng Ma* and add
Shan Zhu Yu (Fructus Corni Officinalis), *Shan Yao* (Radix
Dioscoreae Oppositae), and *Shu Di* (cooked Radix Rehmanniae
Glutinosae).

35. For **qi vacuity fever**, add *Zhi Mu* (Rhizoma Anemarrhenae
Aspheloidis) and *Di Gu Pi* (Cortex Radicis Lycii Chinensis).

36. For **qi vacuity fever**, increase the dosage of *Chai Hu* and add
Huang Qin (Radix Scutellariae Baicalensis) and *Ge Gen* (Radix
Puerariae).

37. For **coronary heart disease with exertional angina pec-
toris** due to concomitant blood stasis, add *Dan Shen* (Radix
Salviae Miltiorrhizae), *Chuan Xiong* (Radix Ligustici Wallichii),
Chi Shao (Radix Rubrus Paeoniae Lactiflorae), *Hong Hua* (Flos
Carthami Tinctorii), and *Jiang Xiang* (Lignum Dalbergiae
Odoriferae).

38. For **chronic sore throat**, add *Jie Geng* (Radix Platycodi
Grandiflori).

39. For **profuse menstruation**, add wine-fried *Bai Shao* (Radix
Albus Paeoniae Lactiflorae). If there is liver heat, also add *Huang
Qin* (Radix Scutellariae Baicalensis).

40. For **flooding and leaking**, add *Di Yu* (Radix Sanguisorbae)
for damp or replete heat, *Ai Ye* (Folium Artemisiae Argyii) and *E
Jiao* (Gelatinum Corii Asini) for qi vacuity, *Sheng Di* (uncooked

Radix Rehmanniae Glutinosae) for vacuity heat, and *Hai Piao Xiao* (Os Sepiae Seu Sepiellae) for loss of securing and astringing.

41. For **profuse menstruation or uterine bleeding** with pale, watery blood accompanied by heart palpitations, shortness of breath, faint, forceless speech, fatigue, and a sagging, dragging feeling in the lower abdomen, subtract *Dang Gui* (Radix Angelicae Sinensis), *Chai Hu* (Radix Bupleuri), and *Chen Pi* (Pericarpium Citri Reticulatae). This results in *Ju Yuan Jian Tang* (Lift the Source Decoction). This formula can then be augmented by adding *Hai Piao Xiao* (Os Sepiae Seu Sepiellae), *Qian Cao* (Radix Rubiae Cordifoliae), and *Wu Mei* (Fructus Pruni Mume). If there is liver heat, also add *Huang Qin* (Radix Scutellariae Baicalensis).

42. For **numbness of the fingers and face** due to qi vacuity with exuberant wind, subtract *Dang Gui, Bai Zhu,* and *Chen Pi* and add *Bai Shao* (Radix Albus Paeoniae Lactiflorae) and *Wu Wei Zi* (Fructus Schisandrae Chinensis).

43. For **numbness accompanying bodily weakness**, dry, flaky skin, and itching, add *Shu Di* (cooked Radix Rehmanniae Glutinosae) and *Bai Shao* (Radix Albus Paeoniae Lactiflorae) to nourish the blood.

44. For concomitant **restlessness of the heart spirit**, add *Long Gu* (Os Draconis), *Mu Li* (Concha Ostreae), and *Ye Jiao Teng* (Caulis Polygoni Multiflori).

Ge Gen Tang (Pueraria Decoction) & *Gui Zhi Tang* (Cinnamon Twig Decoction)

Two other formulas that many famous old Chinese doctors have used extensively beyond their original classical or standard indications are *Ge Gen Tang* (Pueraria Decoction) and *Gui Zhi Tang* (Cinnamon Twig Decoction). Both of these formulas are categorized as acrid, warm, exterior-resolving formulas for the treatment of wind cold exterior contraction in moderate and weak patients respectively. However, it is important to understand that exterior-resolving medicinals are windy-natured, acrid, upbearing medicinals which all out-thrust depression. Therefore, they can also be used to treat liver depression. In fact, *Chai Hu* (Radix Bupleuri), the most commonly used qi-rectifying medicinal is not categorized as a qi-rectifier but as an exterior-resolver. The main ingredient in *Ge Gen Tang* is *Ge Gen* (Radix Puerariae Lobatae), another exterior-resolver. According to Zhuan Yuan,

> *Ge Gen's* flavor is sweet and acrid and its nature is level or neutral. It enters the spleen and stomach channels where its function is to upbear and effuse spleen-stomach clear yang. *It also is able to course and resolve depression and binding of the liver channel's qi mechanism.* [Italics added for emphasis][5]

Because both these formulas also include ingredients to fortify the spleen and supplement the qi as well as to nourish the blood and emolliate the liver, depending on how one modifies them, they may also be used to treat a liver-spleen disharmony. For instance, both formulas include *Bai Shao* (Radix Albus Paeoniae Lactiflorae), *Da Zao* (Fructus Zizyphi Jujubae), mix-fried *Gan Cao* (Radix Glycyrrhizae Uralensis), *Gui Zhi* (Ramulus Cinnamomi Cassiae), and *Sheng Jiang* (uncooked Rhizoma Zingiberis Officinalis). Except for *Gui Zhi*, we have discussed the

> **Once in practice, I encourage practitioners to look deeply into the few most commonly prescribed formulas and attempt to plumb the depth of their functions and indications. When you do this, I feel confident that you will come to see how important the harmonizing formulas are as a basis for the treatment of the majority of our patient population.**

---

[5]Zhuan Yuan, "An Analysis of the Treatment of Middle-aged & Young[Sufferers] of Essential Hypertension by the Methods of Coursing & Rectifying the Liver & Spleen and Regulating & Smoothing the Qi Mechanism," *Shan Dong Zhong Yi Za Zhi (Shandong Journal of Chinese Medicine)*, #5, 2004, p. 265

functions of all these medicinals above. *Gui Zhi* is, in comparison to *Gan Jiang* (dry Rhizoma Zingiberis Officinalis), only mildly warming. It is actually more moving and out-thrusting. It is an excellent medicinal to include in any formula where there are cold hands and/or feet regardless of the other patterns present. *Gui Zhi* also aids the supplementation of the middle qi.

Ge Gen Tang includes *Ge Gen* and *Ma Huang* (Herba Ephedrae). We have seen that *Ge Gen* can also course the liver and rectify the qi. Dr. Zhuan says that, if one puts *Ge Gen* and *Chai Hu* together, "they course and resolve depression and binding in the liver channel and qi mechanism and also upbear and lift the spleen and stomach clear yang."[6] Then, if one deletes *Ma Huang*,[7] one has an excellent base for either adding more spleen-fortifying, qi-supplementing medicinals, more blood-nourishing medicinals, or phlegm-transforming, heat-clearing, qi-rectifying, blood-quickening, or any other kind of medicinals that are necessary for the exigencies of the case at hand. Although I rarely use either of these two formulas in their standard textbook form, I often use them as building blocks as have many other old Chinese doctors before me.

While it is necessary and important to memorize between 80-100 formulas as an undergraduate, it is important to understand that school is different from real-life clinical practice. Once in practice, I encourage practitioners to look deeply into the few most commonly prescribed formulas and attempt to plumb the depth of their functions and indications. When you do this, I feel confident that you will come to see how important the harmonizing formulas are as a basis for the treatment of the majority of our patient population. Further, when we are able to do this, we no longer have to rat through

---

[6]*Ibid.*, p. 265
[7]At this point in time, it is unclear whether or not it is legal for licensed acupuncturists to use *Ma Huang* or not. In decoction, it appears to be legal, but in ready-made formulas it may not be.
[8]*Über* is a German word literally meaning "over," "above," "overarching," or "greater."

this or that book of formulas, nor must we stock such a wide range of medicinals. To me, all the formulas in this chapter and their modifications form one common *über*-formula,[8] any part of which can be combined with any other part. When we understand this, we can also understand why one early 19th century Chinese doctor said, "Medicine is really easy."

Problem Based Learning Exercises (See App. IV for answers)

1. What does harmonizing the liver and spleen mean in clinical practice?

2. What does harmonizing the liver and stomach mean in clinical practice?

3. What does harmonizing the spleen and stomach mean in clinical practice?

4.. What does harmonizing the stomach and intestines mean in clinical practice?

5. What does out-thrusting depression mean?

6. Why are acrid, exterior-resolving medicinals able to course the liver and rectify the qi?

7. What are the treatment principles for a liver-spleen disharmony with stomach heat, phlegm nodulation, and blood stasis resulting in cystic acne? Please write a representative formula.

8. What are the treatment principles for a woman who is premenstrual and presents with a liver-spleen disharmony, stomach heat, and blood vacuity manifesting as fatigue, loose stools, irritability, breast distention and pain, bad breath, and a ravenous appetite? Please write a representative formula.

9. What are the treatment principles for a patient with ulcerative colitis with pus and blood in his stools presenting with a liver-spleen disharmony and damp heat in the intestines? Please write a representative formula.

10. What are the treatment principles for an elderly woman with Sjögren's syndrome who presents with a qi and yin dual vacuity as well as liver depression and blood stasis? Please write a representative formula.

---

[8]*Über* is a German word literally meaning "over," "above," "overarching," or "greater."

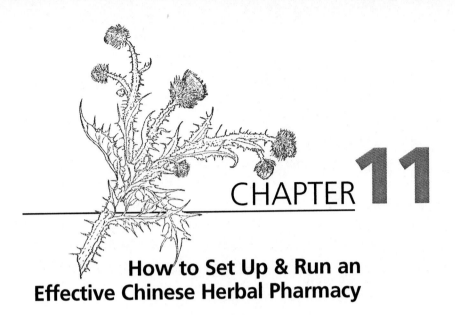

CHAPTER **11**

How to Set Up & Run an Effective Chinese Herbal Pharmacy

Many new practitioners don't set up a pharmacy because they're not sure exactly what to do first. Let's face it, many practitioners may never have had their own business before, and there's a lot to think about when we are first starting out. To make this process a little easier, Honora Lee Wolfe, Marilyn Allen, and Eric Strand tell you pretty much all you need to know (or at least how to find out what you need to know) in their book, *Points for Profit* (also available from Blue Poppy Press). As they point out, it is very difficult to

> **If all we offer is acupuncture, then our income is limited by the number of patients we can see in the number of hours we can work.**

earn a really good living doing acupuncture without also selling your patients something else besides your time. If all we offer is acupuncture, then our income is limited by the number of patients we can see in the number of hours we can work. However, if we also sell our patients other goods and services (which they need and are good for them), then we make a profit on those items as well. In addition, herbal medicines are consumables. That means they are something that the patient must buy over and over again. They are usually not a one-time purchase like a book, tape, or CD (although it's not a bad idea to sell some of those items as well). Setting up an in-house pharmacy or dispensary also has the benefit of providing one-stop shopping for your patients, and, depending upon what lines of products you carry, this may help distinguish you from your competitors.

Starting a ready-made formula dispensary

Unless you feel very confident about your skills writing customized prescriptions, I personally recommend that new practitioners start with a line of ready-made medicines. This is how I started out practicing Chinese herbal medicine. These ready-made medicines can be either Asian-made or American-made. Typically, the Asian-made ready-made pills are very low potency, as we have discussed in other chapters. They are cheap and easy to store, but they also are not very effective for remedial treatment unless dosages are greatly increased from what is written on the bottle. Asian-made extract powders are higher potency. These come in either loose powder form or encapsulated. It is also possible to encapsulate the loose powder yourself on an as-needed basis. Already encapsulated extract powders range in potency from 5:1 to 15:1. Most American-made Chinese herbal pills are also made out of extracts. However, exactly what potency must be determined from your supplier. In any case, I recommend that you start with the following classical formulas which we all studied in school:

1. *Bon Xia Hou Po Tang* (Pinellia and Magnolia bark decoction) Spleen vacuity with dampness and phlegm
2. *Bi Yan Pian* (Rhinitis tablets) Wind heat with phlegm
3. *Bu Zhong Yi Qi Wan* (Supplement the Center & Boost the Qi Pills): Liver-spleen disharmony
4. *Dan Zhi Xiao Yao San* (Moutan & Gardenia Rambling Pills): Liver-spleen disharmony w/blood vacuity & depressive heat
5. *Du Huo Ji Sheng Wan* (Angelica Pubescens & Loranthus Pills): Wind, cold, damp impediment

6. *Er Xian Wan* (Two Immortals Pills): Yin & yang dual vacuity w/ vacuity heat

7. *Er Chen Wan* (Two Aged [Ingredients] Pills): Phlegm dampness

8. *Gui Pi Wan* (Restore the Spleen Pills): Heart-spleen dual vacuity

9. *Huang Lian Jie Du Wan* (Coptis Resolve Toxins Pills): Damp heat, replete heat, heat toxins

10. *Jin Gui Shen Qi Wan* (*Golden Cabinet* Kidney Qi Pills): Kidney yin & yang vacuity

11. *Liu Jun Zi Wan* (Six Gentlemen Pills): Spleen qi vacuity w/ dampness

12. *Liu Wei Di Huang Wan* (Six Flavors Rehmannia Pills): Kidney yin vacuity

13. *Si Jun Zi Wan* (Four Gentlemen Pills): Spleen qi vacuity

14. *Suan Zao Ren Wan* (Zizyphus Spinosa Pills): Liver blood vacuity, vacuity, disquieted spirit

15. *Tian Wang Bu Xin Dan* (Heavenly Emperor Supplement the Heart Elixir): Heart qi & yin vacuity

16. *Wu Ling Wan* (Five [Ingredients] Poria Pills): Water dampness

17. *Xiao Chai Hu Wan* (Minor Bupleurum Pills): Liver-spleen vacuity w/ lung and/or stomach depressive heat

18. *Xiao Yao Wan* (Rambling Pills): Liver-spleen disharmony w/ blood vacuity

19. *Xue Fu Zhu Yu Wan* (Blood Mansion Dispel Stasis Pills): Blood stasis in the chest

20. *Yin Qiao Jie Du Wan* (Lonicera & Forsythia Resolve Toxins Pills): Wind heat external contraction

21. *Zhi Bai Di Huang Wan* (Anemarrhena & Phellodendron Rehmannia Pills): Yin vacuity w/ vacuity heat

In the previous chapter on using only a few basic formulas which you can modify in many ways, I discussed how you can treat many, many patients with combinations of these basic formulas. When you need something for a patient that you don't currently have on your shelf, order it. However, I don't recommend that you order every ready-made medicine in the book just to have on hand "in case." This will tie up too much of your working capital. With FedEx and UPS, you usually can order things as you actually need them, meaning as your patients actually need them, and have them in hand by the next day if necessary. If you buy these formulas in bulk powdered extract form or in encapsulated extract form, they typically come in 100 gram bottles and you could start with as little as one bottle each. If you buy these as ready-made pills, there are usually 12 bottles to a case, and I recommend that you buy a case for two reasons. First, to get the best price, and secondly, because you will probably have to prescribe a higher dose than what's written on the label. Therefore, your patients will go through this type of pill much faster. If you only prescribe and dispense ready-made powder, capsules, and pills by the whole jar or bottle, you can run your dispensary [at least for a while] without hiring a pharmacy worker, even though I do not personally recommend this. (As Marilyn Allen states in *Points for Profit*, it is very difficult to be the caregiver and the person who charges and receives the patient's money. This can be emotionally confusing and embarrassing on both sides.) You will probably be able to store these ready-made medicines without any problem in your current space with your current front desk set-up and clinic storage cabinets.

As your practice gets larger and you understand more about Chinese herbal medicine, you can add more ready-made medicines to your inventory. However, again I recommend that you not buy every ready-made medicine on the market on the off-hand chance that some day you will need it. If you are going to be doing herbs and acupuncture in any case, you can always order a remedy for a patient and have it for the next visit. You may also find that you need higher potency, more complicated ready-made medicines for your patients. Blue Poppy Herbs sells a line of high-potency formulas designed for the most commonly seen multi-pattern disease presentations in Western patients. However, I would not suggest you start with these until you feel that your pattern discrimination has become relatively reliable.

When selling ready-made pills, capsules, and tablets, it is important that they be kept in their original container from the manufacturer. This should have a non-tamper seal and an expiration date plus all the FDA-mandated label information. Do not take pills or tablets out of their original container and count them out into unlabeled baggies. This is unprofessional and potentially illegal.

Starting a singles dispensary

After using ready-made formulas for a while, you will probably become frustrated that there is not always a ready-made formula which exactly matches your patient's needs. At that point you will probably want to put in a singles pharmacy, whether that be powdered extract singles, bulk-dispensed herbs for water decoctions, or alcohol tinctures. Whether you choose powdered extracts or bulk herbs, you will need a scale. I recommend not trying to run a modern pharmacy with the pan and balance scales still used in some traditional Chinese pharmacies. They look cool, but are not the latest technology and not very easy to use! You can buy a good quality electric digital kitchen scale that can weigh in grams or ounces at any good kitchen supply store. You will also need one or more sizes of plastic baggies and one or more sizes of brown paper bags.

The advantages of a powdered extract singles pharmacy include relatively small storage space and good patient compliance. The disadvantages are short shelf life, messy dispensing, and potential high prices to the patient for higher dosage ranges. The advantages of bulk-dispensed herbs are good potency to price (as long as we keep our mark-up reasonable) and longer shelf life. The disadvan-

> The advantages of a powdered extract singles pharmacy include relatively small storage space and good patient compliance. The disadvantages are short shelf life, messy dispensing, and potential high prices to the patient for higher dosage ranges.

tages of bulk-dispensed herbs are the need for separate storage containers, a larger storage area, potentially problematic patient compliance (although I have had few problems with this), quality control, and bugs. Personally, it is my experience that bulk-dispensed, water-based decoctions give you the best price/potency ratio as well as great prescribing flexibility. Therefore, I favor a bulk herb dispensary over a singles extract pharmacy. However, I realize that such a bulk herb dispensary is not right for every patient population, nor for every clinic space, and even I, after drinking Chinese herbal decoctions off and on for 25 plus years, like the ease of extracts when potency, speed, or money are less of an issue.

For powder singles, you may want to purchase a small encapsulation machine. Contact:

1. herbalremedies.com   1-866-467-6444
2. Well Naturally Products (Canada) 1-604-580-3468
3. Capsugel Company   1-888-783-6361
4. Capsuline   1-866-536-2277
   or capsuline.com/pills_filling

As for which herbs to buy first, one way is to make note of the medicinals most commonly used by the mentor whose style you intend to emulate. Then choose 50 of these medicinals for your initial purchase. Many suppliers will give you a one-time special pharmacy set-up discount if you buy enough the first time. In general, the average per pound cost of Chinese herbs whether you are buying 100 grams of extract powder or one pound of bulk is the same: $6.00 per herb. (If there are several different qualities of a single medicinal, I recommend that you buy the medium-priced one.) So the average price of 50 herbs is going to be around $300. With bulk herbs, you will also have to purchase some kind of bottles or containers. Although you can use plastic and that is cheaper, I recommend one gallon glass jars. These will keep your herbs fresher, make a great display for your customers, and retard spoilage and bugs. You can buy this number of glass jars with lids and labels from a local container wholesaler.

You will also need shelf space for these jars, and I definitely recommend that the storage space be visible to your patients. They will love the exotic, old-time apothecary look

> **You should be able to treat the vast majority of patients with 260-300 herbs. In fact, you will find that, most of the time, you are using only around 80-100 ingredients.**

as well as the smell and, if your patients are like mine, will tell their friends about it. Of course, you could also go out and buy or have built a traditional wooden herb cabinet. This is very expensive but can be quite beautiful and will last for years, if not generations!

After you have purchased your initial 50 medicinals, then commit to buying $50 of new herbs per week or per month, depending on your budget until you have a variety of 275-300. This will be in addition to restocking whatever you have used up. If you have a case that requires a specific herb, order it as needed. You should be able to treat the vast majority of patients with 260-300 herbs. In fact, you will find that, most of the time, you are using only around 80-100 ingredients. This is especially so if you specialize, which I very much suggest that you do. I would not stock more than 300 herbs unless you have a case for whom you know you need something. Below are the 82 herbs I would buy first:

Bai Zhu (Rhizoma Atractylodis Macrocephalae)
Bai Shao (Radix Albus Paeoniae Lactiflorae)
Ban Xia (Rhizoma Pinelliae Ternatae)
Cang Zhu (Rhizoma Atractylodis)
Chai Hu (Radix Bupleuri)
Che Qian Zi (Semen Plantaginis)
Chen Pi (Pericarpium Citri Reticulatae)
Chi Shao (Radix Rubrus Paeoniae Lactiflorae)
Chuan Lian Zi (Fructus Meliae Toosendan)

Chuan Xiong (Radix Ligustici Wallichii)
Da Huang (Radix Et Rhizoma Rhei)
Da Zao (Fructus Zizyphi Jujubae)
Dan Pi (Cortex Radicis Moutan)
Dan Shen (Radix Salviae Miltiorrhizae)
Dang Shen (Radix Codonopsitis Pilosulae)
Dang Gui (Radix Angelicae Sinensis)
Du Zhong (Cortex Eucommiae Ulmoidis)
Du Huo (Radix Angelicae Pubescentis)
Fang Feng (Radix Ledebouriellae Divaricatae)
Fu Xiao Mai (Fructus Levis Tritici Aestivi)
Fu Ling (Sclerotium Poriae Cocos)
Gan Jiang (dry Rhizoma Zingiberis Officinalis)
Ge Gen (Radix Puerariae)
Gou Qi Zi (Fructus Lycii Chinensis)
Gou Teng (Ramulus Uncariae Cum Uncis)
Gui Zhi (Ramulus Cinnamomi Cassiae)
Han Lian Cao (Herba Ecliptae Prostratae)
He Huan Pi (Cortex Albizziae Julibrissinis)
He Shou Wu (Radix Polygini Multiflori)
Hong Hua (Flos Carthami Tinctorii)
Hou Po (Cortex Magnoliae Officinalis)
Huang Lian (Rhizoma Coptidis Chinensis)
Huang Qin (Radix Scutellariae Baicalensis)
Huang Qi (Radix Astragali Membranacei)
Huang Bai (Cortex Phellodendri)
Jie Geng (Radix Platycodi Grandiflori)
Jin Yin Hua (Flos Lonicerae Japonicae)
Lian Qiao (Fructus Forsythiae Suspensae)
Long Gu (Os Draconis)
Mai Ya (Fructus Germinatus Hordei Vulgaris)
Mai Men Dong (Tuber Ophiopogonis Japonici)
mix-fried *Gan Cao* (Radix Glycyrrhizae Uralensis)
Mu Tong (Caulis Akebiae)
Mu Li (Concha Ostreae)
Mu Xiang (Radix Auklandiae Lappae)
Niu Xi (Radix Achyranthis Bidentatae)

Nu Zhen Zi (Fructus Ligustri Lucidi)

Pu Gong Ying (Herba Taraxaci Mongolici)

Qiang Huo (Radix Et Rhizoma Notopterygii)

Rou Gui (Cortex Cinnamomi Cassiae)

San Qi (Radix Pseudoginseng)

Sang Ji Sheng (Ramulus Loranthi Seu Visci)

Sha Ren (Fructus Amomi)

Shan Zhu Yu (Fructus Corni Officinalis)

Shan Zha (Fructus Crataegi)

Shan Yao (Radix Dioscoreae Oppositae)

Sheng Di (uncooked Radix Rehmanniae Glutinosae)

Sheng Jiang (uncooked Rhizoma Zingiberis Officinalis)

Shi Chang Pu (Rhizoma Acori Graminei)

Shi Jue Ming (Concha Haliotidis)

Shu Di (cooked Radix Rehmanniae Glutinosae)

Suan Zao Ren (Semen Zizyphi Jujubae)

Tao Ren (Semen Pruni Persicae)

Tian Hua Fen (Radix Trichosanthis Kirlowii)

Tu Si Zi (Semen Cuscutae Chinensis)

uncooked *Gan Cao* (Radix Glycyrrhizae Uralensis)

Wei Ling Xian (Radix Clematidis Chinensis)

Wu Wei Zi (Fructus Schisandrae Chinensis)

Wu Mei (Fructus Pruni Mume)

Xiang Fu (Rhizoma Cyperi Rotundi)

Xing Ren (Semen Pruni Armeniacae)

Xu Duan (Radix Dipsaci)

Yan Hu Suo (Rhizoma Corydalis Yanhusuo)

Ye Jiao Teng (Caulis Polygonis Multiflori)

Yi Yi Ren (Semen Coicis Lachryma-jobi)

Yu Jin (Tuber Curcumae)

Yuan Zhi (Rhizoma Polygalae Tenuifoliae)

Ze Xie (Rhizoma Alismatis Orientalis)

Zhe Bei Mu (Bulbus Fritillariae Thunbergii)

Zhi Ke (Fructus Citri Aurantii)

Zhi Shi (Fructus Immaturus Citri Aurantii)

Zhi Zi (Fructus Gardeniae Jasminoidis)

Zhu Ru (Caulis Bambusae In Taeniis)

Once you decide to bite the bullet and have a singles pharmacy and write and fill your own prescriptions in-house, the next thing you need to do is hire a helper. Most every practitioner balks at taking this step at first—as did I as a young practitioner. But think about it: you can earn $60-100 or more per hour seeing patients. You should be able to hire a pharmacy helper for $9-12 per hour. If you try to see patients and make their formulas up, it will take away from the number of patients you can see. Do you want to pay yourself $10 per hour or $100? It's simple mathematics. Unless you are only seeing a few people per week, *you cannot afford to make up your patients' herbal formulas yourself.* The good news is that this helper will be able to free up your time in a lot of other ways. He or she can answer the phone, schedule appointments, do your basic book-keeping and filing, do your purchasing, keep your inventories, and, most importantly, tell your patients what they owe and collect the money. It is not likely that you will keep your dispensary person busy full time just making up formulas. Therefore, he or she can also be your front desk person, and, no matter what, at some point fairly early in your practice, it is my belief that you absolutely have to have a front desk person. A front desk person is one of the main things that will make the difference between subsistence earnings and having a going commercial concern.

> **A front desk person is one of the main things that will make the difference between subsistence earnings and having a going commercial concern. Having your front desk person also make up prescriptions will keep them busy and actually help pay for their salary.**

Having your front desk person also make up prescriptions will keep them busy and actually help pay for their salary.

Although I know people who have single dispensaries in alcohol tincture form, I have no experience with this myself. Nevertheless, the herbs that I would stock first would be the same. The measuring out of formulas would be by some fluid measurement as opposed to weight, and you would need to buy small bottles and dropper caps for the custom-blended formulas to be put in. Clear or amber-colored, dropper bottles are available from wholesale packaging supply houses.

If you choose to dispense either powdered extract or tinctured formulas, you can usually include dosage and administration instructions on the label, which you could also make yourself on a laser printer. If you put your clinic name and phone number, such labels are even good marketing. However, if you choose to dispense bulk herbs for decoction, you will need to create a printed instruction sheet explaining to the patient as clearly and simply as possible how to make and take their decoction. In my experience, it is possible to create a single-sided sheet with check boxes that can work with any formula and dosage regimen. (There is a sample form included in Appendix III.) For instance, there can be several check boxes for cooking time of the main herbs. Then there can be check boxes for precooked, short-cooked, steeped, and dissolved medicinals.

You, as the prescribing practitioner, should fill out this form which is then passed to your dispensary helper along with the actual prescription to be made up. When the patient comes to pick up their formula, these printed instructions should be included in the bag with the herbs. For first-time patients, the dispensary helper should read the instructions to the patient, explain anything the patient needs explained, and ask if the patient has any questions. Since efficacy from Chinese herbal decoctions partially depends on correct cooking, it is important that the patient understands exactly what he or she is supposed to do. As yet another source of collateral income, you might also sell Chinese herb cooking pots in your clinic. These are inexpensive, are designed and dedicated to this single purpose, and are another way to provide one-stop shopping for your patients.

What to charge
Many practitioners have a hard time figuring out what to

charge for their herbal remedies, whether these be ready-made or custom-filled. I have seen practitioners charge both too much and too little. What you charge should not be pulled from out of the air, but rather be based on sound business mathematics. If you are selling ready-made medicines, you should double their price if they are cheaper, Asian-made medicines. If they are more expensive U.S.-made medicines, you should mark them up at least 50% above what they cost you. (Don't forget to include the shipping cost when determining what the medicinal costs you.) Such markups are fair, reasonable, and standard. After all, we would not expect a shoe store, a food store, or a restaurant not to mark up their products and our businesses are the same. Anything that takes up space and cash flow needs to bring in at least some amount of profit or we cannot afford to sell it!

When it comes to custom-filled formulas, some clinics have a set price per formula no matter whether the ingredients are expensive or cheap and whether there are only a few or more than 20 ingredients in the formula. The idea is that, on average, the clinic will make money. When doing it this way, there is the tendency to charge whatever the market will bear because one does not want to lose money on the transaction. However, there is another way to do it that I personally think is more equitable for everyone.

Figure out the per gram cost of each ingredient. This can then be entered into a computerized program or into a hard-copy ledger. If we know that there are 16 ounces to a pound and 28 grams to an ounce, this is fairly straightforward. Then figure out the percentage of markup you would like to make on your single herbs. This can be anywhere from 50-100%. Add this markup to the per gram cost listed in your ledger. When the dispensary person fills the prescription, they figure out exactly what the prescription should actually cost. Next they figure in the cost of any supplies, such as plastic baggies and brown paper bags. Then they take the time they spent making the formula, divide that part of an hour into their hourly wage and add all this together. *Violá*. You *know* that you are making money on each and every prescription filled, and the patient knows that they are paying a fair and equitable price for their medicine.

Figuring the Cost for Bulk Prescriptions

Price per gram including percentage of markup x number of grams per ingredient

+ cost of plastic baggies
+ cost of brown paper bag
+ cost of time to make Rx
= cost of patient's medicine

This same equation can also be used to price custom-blended alcohol tinctures. However, in that case, you will have to substitute ounces or drams for grams and bottles for baggies. Otherwise, everything is the same.

While it will take your herb dispensary/front desk person a little time to learn the per gram prices, with a little practice, he or she will not have to look at the book or even use the computerized system. With a little practice, they will also become very quick at weighing out each medicinal. Our herb dispensary person has been doing her job for so long that she can tell you when she has 9-10 grams of all the most commonly used medicinals just by the way it feels or fills her hand. Over time, she has also learned how to tell good quality from bad quality of all the major ingredients and knows when something doesn't look, feel, or smell right. It takes her only 2-3 minutes to do the math for a given prescription.

Returns
Every now and again, for whatever reason, a patient will ask if

he or she can return some or all of their medicine. Of course it's not a problem to accept returns of any ready-made medicines that are unopened. We do not accept returns of any ready-made medicine that has been opened and I don't feel that you should do so either. Individually written and filled extract powder formulas should also not be returnable since the powders can not be separated out again. At our clinic, we do allow returns of bulk-filled prescriptions under the following conditions: We will credit the patient's account for 50% the per gram price of any ingredients that can be easily separated by our pharmacy staff. Any ingredients that cannot be separated are not returnable. We insist that the separation be done by our clinic staff wearing clean plastic gloves. Patients must be made to understand that this is a compromise solution for both parties. Given the nature of bulk-filled prescriptions, this is the best one can do.

> **Once you have a singles dispensary, be it powdered extracts, alcohol tinctures, or bulk herbs, you will very likely wonder how you ever got along without one.**

Conclusion

Once you have a singles dispensary, be it powdered extracts, alcohol tinctures, or bulk herbs, you will very likely wonder how you ever got along without one. It will be a great source of extra revenue, it will help pay for clinic support staff, and should improve your therapeutic outcomes—all great reasons to move in this direction. However, you will still want to keep a selection of ready-made Chinese medicines in your clinic. There will always be cases where such ready-made medicines provide a simple, cost-effective solution for the patient. In fact, after you've been prescribing complex customized formulas, you may appreciate all the more the high-potency, complex ready-made formulas such as the ones Blue Poppy Herbs offers.

Problem Based Learning Exercises (See App. IV for answers)

1. Contact several Chinese herb suppliers and find out the cost of one case of each of the Chinese herbal formulas you would like to initially stock will cost. Ask them for an initial dispensary start-up discount.

2. Write a representative formula for a hypothetical patient. If you plan on selling custom-blended formulas from powdered extracts, find out how much 100 grams of each of the ingredients would be. Then add your markup and figure out the selling price of that formula to your patient. If you plan on having a bulk herb pharmacy, cost out the formula the same way. If you plan on hiring an herbal dispensary helper, figure a portion of their hourly wage to the final cost. Also figure in the cost of plastic baggies and paper bags.

3. On page 142 is a suggested ready-made medicines "starter" list. Divide this list into categories by function (exterior-resolvers, qi supplements, blood quickeners, etc.). Are there other ready-made formulas that you feel you need? Add those to your list as needed. By calling several companies, find out what creating this initial pharmacy will cost.

4. Find out the "footprint" or dimensions of the jars you plan on using for either powdered extracts or bulk herbs. Then calculate the number and size of shelves you will need to store these ingredients. Consider whether you will build the shelving yourself or have it professionally built. If you intend on building the shelves yourself, find out how much the materials will cost. If you are going to have the shelving built, get an estimate from a carpenter. Also consider the footprint of the shelving and any herbal formula preparation area and what fraction of your clinic's square footage that will be. Then figure in the cost of that square footage into what income your dispensary must generate per month/year.

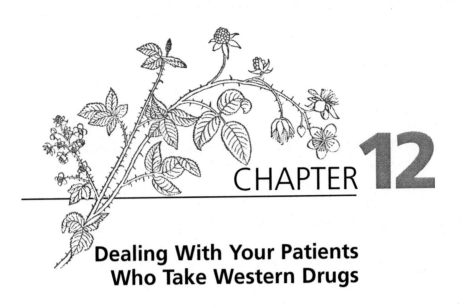

CHAPTER 12

Dealing With Your Patients Who Take Western Drugs

As our patient population continues to age, more and more of them are taking one or more Western medications. Therefore, an increasingly common question is what to do in terms of Chinese herbal medicine when patients are concurrently using Western meds. Unfortunately, there is no single easy answer for this question. We are dealing with a historical situation that Chinese medicine has never dealt with before, and it is unlikely in our lifetime that we will have all the definitive answers to this question that we would like to have. That being said, there are some things about this situation that we can say.

First, you can choose simply not to prescribe Chinese herbal medicines to patients on Western meds. In that case, you can attempt to treat them with acupuncture, moxibustion, tuina, and other related external therapies alone. There is no rule that says that all patients need to be treated with acupuncture *and* Chinese medicinals. In fact, the norm in China is for acupuncturists to only treat with acupuncture, and for internal Chinese medical practitioners to only treat with Chinese herbs. Further, such a decision does not have to be irrevocable. I have often told patients on discretionary Western medications, such as oral contraceptives or HRT (hormone replacement therapy) that, if they ever decide to stop taking the Western meds in question, either because they don't work or they have too many side effects, I would be happy to try to treat them with internally administered Chinese herbal medicinals. While taking this route eliminates any worry about possible herb-drug interactions, it may unacceptably limit one's potential patient population.

Secondly, you can choose to prescribe Chinese medicinals at the same time as the patient is taking Western meds prescribed by one or more Western physicians. In that case:

1. Be sure to find out all of the Western medications the patient is taking and their doses. Then go to a Western medical source, such as *The Essential Guide to Prescription Drugs*, and read up about each medication. If possible, also attempt to work out provisional Chinese medical descriptions for these drugs. For example, does this drug function as a heat clearer, a surface resolver, a qi supplement, or what? This is knowable (at least to a large extent) by looking at both the intended therapeutic effect as well as the unwanted side effects.

2. Determine from the patient if the Western meds are A) achieving their intended therapeutic effect satisfactorily and B) whether they are causing any side effects.

A. If one or more Western meds are not achieving their intended effect, we have to consider whether each Western medication is appropriate for our patient's personally presenting pattern based on that medication's provisional Chinese medical prescription. For instance, Clomid®, a fertility drug which stimulates ovulation, is clearly a yang-invigorating, kidney-supplementing medicinal which can cause yin vacuity/vacuity heat in patient's who are predisposed to yin vacuity. In that case, I would not prescribe any more yang supplements but rather yin supplements and vacuity heat-clearing medicinals to moderate or "harmonize" the effects of the Clomid® for that particular patient.

B. If one or more Western meds are achieving their intended therapeutic effect but are causing side effects in the process, then I would not prescribe duplicate Chinese meds to achieve that same intended therapeutic effect. Rather I would prescribe Chinese medicinals based on the patient's presenting patterns including the side effects. In this case, the goal is to allow the Western medication(s) to continue doing their job while eliminating any side effects.

3. After determining what Chinese medicinals you would like to prescribe, go to one or more sources to research if there are any known drug interactions between the patient's Western meds and those Chinese medicinals. Blue Poppy Press's *Herb Toxicities & Drug Interactions*, by Fred Jennes is just such a source. If there are any known drug interactions between what you would like to prescribe and what the patient is already taking, then you should consider either A) leaving that ingredient out of your formula, B) substituting another Chinese medicinal for that ingredient, C) reducing that ingredient's dose, and/or D) adding one or more ingredients to prevent such a reaction. This last suggestion is possible only if we can work out the Chinese medical mechanisms for the interaction, and this may not be possible. Therefore, this last possibility is the least likely of our choices.

4. Once I have decided on my Chinese herbal formula and feel reasonably sure that it is not likely to cause any drug-interactions, I begin by *carefully* starting the patient off with a small trial dose. By this, I mean to keep the dosages of the individual Chinese medicinals on the small side as well as to only give the patient a couple of days worth of

herbs. For instance, I routinely start my patients out on a four-day dose. At the end of that time, I tell them to call me to let me know how they did. If they have had any side effects, this allows me to immediately change their prescription before too much damage has been done. In some cases, I may ask patients to call me after only a single day or two days. If the prescription has not caused any problems or adverse reactions, I then prescribe a one week's dose. At the end of that time, again the patient calls in to tell me how they are doing, and again I prescribe another week's dose or, if they are doing really well, I may prescribe as much as two weeks' dose at a time. However, I make sure that the patient stays in touch with me on a regular basis so that, if any problems crop up, I can immediately solve those problems as necessary. Further, I make sure the patient knows what I consider a problem. Depending on the herbs and their Western meds, that may mean sleep disturbances, digestive complaints, skin rashes, or whatever. At the time, I try to assure the patient that these reactions are *not* expected—that they are unlikely. However, in the unlikely event that one of them does occur, I want to know ASAP.

5. If possible, open a dialogue with the prescribing Western physician(s). Some will simply not want to talk. Others will talk but not really listen. Some will forbid their patients to take any Chinese herbs while taking their Western meds for fear of some unknown herb-drug interaction. In that case, there may not be much you can do. If possible, consider sending them a copy of Fred Jennes's book *Herb Toxicities & Drug Interactions* to show them that you diligently study the available literature on this subject and act responsibly. If possible, also send the physician copies of any research reports or pages from Chinese medical books which show that, in general, the combination of Chinese and Western meds in the disease at hand are safe.

Bottom line, everything in the Chinese medical literature suggests that Chinese medicinals *correctly prescribed on the basis of the patient's personally presenting patterns* are generally safe when taken in tandem with most Western drugs. In China today, most Chinese use Western medicine. Only 25% use Chinese medicine and even these do not necessarily use Chinese medicine exclusively. That means that many, many Chinese (potentially millions) are routinely treated with both Chinese and Western medications. I read the Chinese medical literature assiduously looking specifically for articles on herb-drug interactions since I know there is currently so much concern over this issue. However, reports of such interactions are almost nil, and I have to think that more articles would be published about this if such interactions were common. Over the last five years, I have worked on a half-dozen big books having to do with the Chinese medical treatment of this or that Western medical specialty, such as diabetes, nephrology, psychiatry, and cardiology. In doing the research for those books, I have read and translated hundreds upon hundreds of Chinese journal articles, many of them discussing case histories or clinical trials where patients were treated with a combination of Chinese and Western medicine, so-called integrated Chinese-Western medicine. What I can say from all this recent research is that the combination of Chinese and Western medicines appears to achieve better therapeutic effects at smaller dosages of the Western drugs and with less or no side effects. This means that, if anything, the combination of modern Western and traditional Chinese medicines is a good thing, not something to be feared, avoided, or forbidden. Based on my 25 plus years of clinical experience, I believe that, if one proceeds carefully and with due diligence, there is little danger of herb-drug interactions.

APPENDIX I

What's Wrong With the Term "Patent Medicines"?

Most acupuncturists and practitioners of Chinese medicine in the West refer to ready-made Chinese medicines (*cheng zhong yao*) as "patent medicines." That is the word most of us were taught in school. For years now I have been arguing against our use of this term. Not only is it factually inaccurate, it also stigmatizes our medicines in the eyes of those who actually know what patent medicines are. The following is a definition of patent medicines I found on the Web:

> The words "patent medicine" refer to products that were marketed, mostly in the 19th century, as medicines that would cure a host of diseases. Many of the diseases which these medicines were supposed to cure are still not curable today—cancer and diabetes, for example. Why did people buy these products? Well, given that the access to medical practitioners was limited, especially in rural areas, and the state of medical technology in the 19th century, who wouldn't buy these products? After all, going to your general store and purchasing a prepared medicine was a lot easier and a lot more pleasant than going to a doctor and having him perform bloodletting![1]

In other words, "patent medicines" refer to 19th century

---

[1]www.cyberus.ca/~sjordan/pmhist.htm

> **In other words, "patent medicines" refer to 19th century "snake oil," and the use of this term plays directly into the hands of those who would denigrate our medicine as quackery.**

"snake oil," and the use of this term plays directly into the hands of those who would denigrate our medicine as quackery. Why were these 19th century ready-made medicines called patent medicines? The explanation is given by the same e-source:

> In mid-18th century England, some producers of medical preparations applied for and obtained Royal Patents for their products. The patents protected the owners' rights to the products and gave some prestige to the medicines. Robert Turlington was one of the very first to receive a Royal Patent for his "Balsam of Life." Later on, the term patent medicine was applied to any of this type of product, whether patented or not.[2]

The fact that this term is pejorative and detrimental to the public perception of our medicine is aptly demonstrated by the following FDA page on patent medicines published under the title, "The Patent Medicine Menace." Because it is the "official" U.S. governmental position on patent medicines, I am presenting it here in its entirety. I hope it serves as a wake-up call to our profession to stop using this archaic, inaccurate, and defamatory term.

> Patent medicines have had a long and ignominious history in the U.S., reaching their zenith in the late 19th century. As the population became more urban and somewhat more capitalized, a ripe target emerged for some post-industrial entrepreneurs, entrepreneurs who would thrive in a marketplace best characterized by the dictum, 'caveat emptor.' Communications had expanded, and the printed word became a crucial venue for the proliferation of patent medicines. The rise of advertising in America, not coincidentally, paralleled the rise of nostrums. At the same time, the biomedical sciences in this country were still in their infancy, and medicine was ill-equipped to deal with

---

[2]*Ibid.*

most diseases. An army of enterprising individuals were prepared to step in and alleviate the suffering.

Nostrums permeated American society by the late 19th century. Products appealed to exotica, the medical knowledge of Native Americans, death, religion, patriotism, mythology (a natural for this industry!), and especially new developments in science. There was nothing to stop patent medicine makers from claiming anything and putting anything in their products, clearly seen in the famous morphine and alcohol-laced soothing syrups for teething and colicky babies. Cancer and arthritis cures, baldness remedies, bust developers, manhood restorers—wherever a need existed, patent medicine makers stepped in. They did not have a monopoly on the market, though. The ethical pharmaceutical industry, those firms that advertised for the most part directly to health professionals, sold their share of nostrums as well.

Quacks developed successful marketing techniques, but they also promoted their interests in more surreptitious ways. For example, they subdued any curiosity in the press with their economic strength. By the 1890s, patent medicine manufacturers used so-called "red clauses" in their advertising contracts with newspapers and magazines. These muzzle clauses voided the contract if state laws regulating nostrums were passed. Thus, not only were many editorials silent on the need for such laws, they actively campaigned against them.

But quacks and their trade associations were not able to stifle the entire fourth estate. A few muckraking journalists helped expose the red clauses, the false testimonials, the nostrums laden with harmful ingredients, the unfounded cures for cancer, tuberculosis, syphilis, narcotic addiction, and a host of other serious as well as self-limited diseases. The most influential work in this genre was the series by Samuel Hopkins Adams that appeared in *Collier's* on October 7, 1905, titled "The Great American Fraud." Adams published 10 articles in the series which concluded in February 1906. He followed this up with another series on doctors who advertised fake clinics. The shocking stories of the patent medicine menace were accompanied by startling images, such as "Death's Laboratory."

That same month saw the publication of another work which,

more than any other single event, spurred on passage of the 1906 act. Socialist writer Upton Sinclair published *The Jungle*, a fact-based novel about immigrant life in the meat-packing industry of Chicago. Sinclair's shocking and revolting story, verified by government undercover investigators, primed the final push for a federal law.

The first federal Food and Drugs Act was passed four months later. The exposés of muckrakers like Adams and Sinclair had a major impact on passage of the bill, as did the untiring work of the General Federation of Women's Clubs, state food and drug officials, the American Medical Association, and the American Pharmaceutical Association. Most notable among the reformers was the head of the Bureau of Chemistry of the U. S. Department of Agriculture, Harvey Washington Wiley, who stumped for remedial legislation since his arrival in Washington in 1883 (though Wiley was much more concerned with food supply). The law prohibited adulteration and misbranding of food and drugs, and though it had many shortcomings, it was arguably the pinnacle of Progressive Era legislation. It did not put quackery out of business; that still thrives. But it brought some disclosure and accountability into the marketplace, an important first step in consumer protection.[3]

At this point in time, Chinese herbal medicine is experiencing an image problem. There have been the deaths from kidney failure in Europe and the U.S. due to aristolochic acid, there has been the discovery and broadcasting of the adulteration of a number of Chinese ready-made medicines with Western scheduled drugs, and, most recently, there has been the FDA banning of *Ma Huang* (Herba Ephedrae) and *Ban Xia* (Rhizoma Pinelliae Ternatae) from all dietary supplements. As the FDA has made clear in public communications, if this last ban is made to stick, it plans to ban other substances from dietary supplements, including all of the citrus family of herbs, such as *Chen Pi* (Pericarpium Citri Reticulatae), *Qing Pi* (Pericarpium Citri Reticulatae Viride), *Zhi Ke* (Fructus Citri Aurantii), *Zhi Shi* (Fructus Immaturus Citri Aurantii), and *Fo Shou* (Fructus Citri Sacrodactylis), due to these herbs' inclu-

---

[3]www.fda.gov/cder/about/history/gallery/galleryintro.htm

sion of the medically active ingredient sinephrine. Ready-made Chinese medicines sold in the U.S. are done so legally as "dietary supplements" under DSHEA (the Dietary Supplement & Health Education Act) even though, in actuality, that is not what they are. At the moment, we need all the good press and PR we can get. Therefore, I believe we should immediately jettison our use of the term "patent medicine" and switch to the direct English translation of what these medicines are called in Chinese, *cheng zhong yao*, prepared or ready-made Chinese medicines.

Ready-made Chinese medicines includes all those Chinese medicines which are available in ready-made form, such as pills, capsules, tablets, powdered extracts, tinctures, medicated oils, and plasters, whether made in Asia or in the West. Several years ago, the government of the People's Republic of China realized that ready-made Chinese herbal medicines had a problem with perceived quality. Currently, quality control is job #1 of the Chinese medical division of the SDA, the State Drug Administration, China's equivalent of the FDA.

The Chinese herbal business represents $25 billion dollars per year of income to the PRC, mostly in hard currencies from countries such as the U.S., Germany, and Canada. In fact, the U.S. accounts for 15% of this total, more than domestic Chinese sales. So the U.S. market is extremely important to the leaders of the PRC, and they are doing everything they can to insure that access to this cash cow is well protected. For instance, by governmental fiat, all Chinese drug manufactures must be Good Manufacturing Practice (GMP)-certified by the end of 2004, and China will be the first country in the world to institute Good Agricultural Procedures (GAP, 2007) which have been specifically designed for the Chinese herbal industry.

Further, American distributors and manufacturers of ready-made Chinese medicines have taken great strides in the last several years to insure quality control on this end. These companies now routinely require testing on every batch of every medicine with set standards for microbial, heavy metal, and pesticide residue contamination. In addition, all these American companies will be required by the U.S. FDA in the near future to comply with GMPs, and already all companies selling ready-made Chinese medicinals in the U.S. must meet FDA labeling standards for herb identifications, etc. on their packaging.

> **I believe that, in order for this medicine to survive in an increasingly hostile regulatory environment, we, as a profession, need to make a concerted effort to abandon this out-dated and pejorative label and switch to the more correct and neutral term of prepared or ready-made Chinese medicines.**

The point that I am trying to make is that the ready-made Chinese medicine industry in the U.S., China, and Taiwan has greatly improved quality control over even just five years ago. However, both prescribers (us) and consumers (patients) continue to foster a false perception of the poor and even dangerous quality of these products when we erroneously refer to them as "patent medicines." I believe that, in order for this medicine to survive in an increasingly hostile regulatory environment, we, as a profession, need to make a concerted effort to abandon this out-dated and pejorative label and switch to the more correct and neutral term of prepared or ready-made Chinese medicines. If we continue using this out-dated and incorrect word to describe one of the most important parts of our practice here in the West, we will, ourselves, be at least partially to blame when the FDA attempts to regulate us out of business.

APPENDIX II

Treatment Principles
Correlated to Patterns

Qi vacuity: Supplement the qi

Blood vacuity: Either supplement or nourish the blood

Yin vacuity: Either supplement, nourish, or enrich yin

Yang vacuity: Either supplement, warm, or invigorate yang

Yang desertion: Rescue yang and stem desertion

Yin desertion: Nourish qi and yin, stem desertion

Qi desertion: Greatly supplement the qi, return yang, and stem desertion

Blood desertion: Supplement the qi and stem desertion

Blood vacuity: Nourish or supplement and regulate the blood

Blood stasis: Quicken the blood and transform or dispel stasis

Blood stasis in the network vessels: Quicken the blood and
   free the flow or open the network vessels

Blood heat: Clear heat, cool the blood, and stop bleeding

Phlegm rheum: Warm and transform phlegm rheum, fortify the
   spleen and disinhibit dampness

Phlegm dampness: Transform phlegm and dry dampness, rectify
   the qi and harmonize the center

Phlegm nodulation or binding: Transform phlegm, scatter
   nodulation or binding, and/or soften the hard

Damp heat: Clear heat and eliminate dampness

Heat toxins: Clear heat and resolve toxins

Wind striking the channels and network vessels: Dispel wind and free the flow of the channels

Dampness striking the channels and network vessels: Eliminate dampness and free the flow of the channels

Cold striking the channels and network vessels: Warm the channels and scatter cold

Wind damp impediment: Dispel wind and eliminate dampness, free the flow of impediment and stop pain

Damp heat impediment: Clear heat and eliminate dampness, free the flow of impediment and stop pain

Cough: Stop coughing

Panting: Stop, level, or stabilize panting

Diarrhea: Stop diarrhea

Dysentery: Stop dysentery

Bleeding: Stop bleeding

Vomiting: Stop vomiting

Sweating: Stop sweating

Pain: Stop or stabilize pain

Tetany: Stop tetany

Irregular menstruation: Regulate the menses

Restless fetal stirring: Quiet the fetus

Constipation: Free the flow of the stools

Strangury: Free the flow of strangury

Disquieted spirit: Quiet, calm, still, and/or settle the spirit

Insomnia: Quiet the sleep

Syncope: Arouse the spirit

Summerheat: Clear summerheat

Summerheat heat: Clear summerheat and drain fire

Summerheat dampness: Clear summerheat and eliminate dampness

Dampness: Eliminate, transform, dry, seep, or disinhibit dampness

Dryness: Moisten dryness and/or engender fluids

Exterior contraction: Resolve the exterior

Interior repletion: Drain the interior

Interior cold: Warm the interior

Externally contracted wind: Course or dispel wind

Internally engendered wind: Extinguish or track down wind

Liver depression qi stagnation: Course the liver and rectify
the qi

Liver-spleen disharmony: Harmonize the liver and spleen

Liver-stomach disharmony: Harmonize the liver and stomach

Liver depression-depressive or transformative heat: Course the liver
and rectify the qi, resolve depression and clear heat

Liver-stomach depressive heat: Clear the liver and stomach, resolve
depression and downbear counterflow or harmonize the stomach

Liver depression and blood vacuity: Harmonize the liver

Ascendant liver yang hyperactivity: Clear the liver and subdue yang
or subdue yang and downbear counterflow

Upward flaming of liver fire: Clear the liver and drain fire

Internal stirring of liver wind: Settle the liver and extinguish wind

Liver blood insufficiency or vacuity: Relax or emolliate the liver and
nourish the blood

Liver blood-kidney yin vacuity: Nourish the liver and enrich the
kidneys

Liver blood-kidney yang vacuity: Nourish the liver and supplement
the kidneys, warm and invigorate yang

Yin vacuity-yang hyperactivity: Enrich yin and subdue yang

Liver-gallbladder damp heat: Clear heat and eliminate dampness from
the liver and gallbladder

Cold stagnating in the liver vessels: Warm the liver and scatter cold,
rectify the qi and stop pain

Heart qi vacuity: Supplement the heart qi

Heart blood vacuity: Supplement heart blood

Heart yin vacuity: Supplement heart yin

Heart yang vacuity: Supplement the heart and warm yang

Heart-spleen dual vacuity: Fortify the spleen and nourish the heart, supplement the qi and blood

Heart-gallbladder qi vacuity: Fortify the spleen and nourish the heart, transform phlegm and rectify the qi

Heart fire effulgence: Clear the heart and drain fire

Phlegm confounding the heart orifices: Transform phlegm and open the orifices

Phlegm fire harassing the heart: Transform phlegm and drain fire, clear the liver and settle the heart

Heart blood stasis: Quicken the blood and dispel stasis

Heart and kidneys not interacting (with yang vacuity below): Clear the heart and lead yang to move downward

Heart and kidneys not interacting (with yin vacuity below): Clear the heart and enrich the kidneys, promote the interaction of above and below

Heart fire transmitted to the small intestine: Clear heat and enrich yin, disinhibit water and free the flow of strangury

Spleen qi vacuity: Fortify the spleen and supplement or boost the qi

Spleen qi downward fall: Fortify the spleen, boost the qi, and lift the fallen

Spleen vacuity with stomach heat: Fortify the spleen and clear the stomach and/or harmonize the center

Spleen yang vacuity: Warm the spleen and supplement the qi

Spleen-kidney yang vacuity: Fortify the spleen and boost the qi, supplement the kidneys and invigorate yang

Spleen vacuity with damp encumbrance: Fortify the spleen and eliminate dampness

Damp heat smoldering in the spleen: Clear heat and disinhibit dampness

Food stagnation in the stomach duct: Disperse accumulation and/or abduct stagnation

Stomach qi counterflowing upward: Harmonize the stomach and/or downbear counterflow

Stomach fire effulgence: Clear the stomach and drain fire

Stomach heat and yin vacuity: Clear the stomach and nourish yin or engender fluids

Stomach yin vacuity with damp heat: Clear heat and eliminate dampness, nourish the stomach and rectify the qi

Stomach yin vacuity: Nourish the yin and stomach, rectify the qi and engender fluids

Stomach blood stasis: Quicken the blood and transform stasis

Wind cold raiding the lungs: Course wind and scatter cold, diffuse the lungs and stop coughing

Wind heat attacking the lungs: Course wind and clear heat, diffuse the lungs and transform phlegm

Wind dryness damaging the lungs: Course wind and clear the lungs, moisten dryness and stop coughing

Summerheat damaging the lungs network vessels: Clear heat and resolve toxins, cool the blood and stop bleeding

Phlegm heat depressing the lungs: Transform phlegm and clear heat, loosen the chest and resolve depression

Lung heat smoldering and exuberance: Clear the lungs and drain fire

Damp heat smoldering in the lungs: Clear the lungs and eliminate dampness, dispel stasis and discharge pus

Phlegm turbidity obstructing the lungs: Transform phlegm and dry dampness, fortify the spleen and stop coughing

Lung qi vacuity: Supplement the lungs and boost the qi

Lung-spleen dual vacuity: Fortify the spleen and boost the qi, supplement earth to engender metal

Cold rheum hidden in the lungs: Warm and transform cold rheum

Lung qi vacuity with simultaneous heat: Supplement the qi and clear heat, transform phlegm and stop coughing

Lung dryness with simultaneous phlegm: Moisten the lungs and clear heat, rectify the qi and transform phlegm

Lung yin vacuity: Enrich yin and moisten the lungs

Lung qi and yin dual vacuity: Clear heat and moisten dryness, supplement the qi and nourish yin

Lung qi and yin dual vacuity with phlegm heat: Moisten the lungs and supplement the qi, clear heat and transform phlegm

Lung-kidney yin vacuity: Supplement the kidneys and moisten the lungs, transform phlegm and stop coughing

Lung-kidney yang vacuity: Supplement the lungs and promote the absorption of the qi, downbear the qi and stabilize panting

Lung network vessel stasis and obstruction: Quicken the blood and transform stasis, free the flow of the network vessels and stop bleeding

Large intestine heat accumulation: Precipitate and discharge heat and accumulation from the large intestine, free the flow of the stools

Large intestine damp heat: Clear heat, transform dampness, and free the flow of the stools

Large intestine fluid dryness: Nourish the blood, moisten dryness, and free the flow of the stools

Large intestine heat stasis: Clear heat and disinhibit dampness, quicken the blood and dispel stasis

Kidney qi vacuity: Supplement the kidneys and boost the qi

Kidneys not securing the essence: Supplement the kidneys and secure the essence

Kidneys not securing and astringing the intestines: Warm and supplement the kidneys, astringe the intestines and stop diarrhea

Kidneys not absorbing the qi: Supplement the kidneys to absorb the qi

Kidney yang vacuity: Supplement the kidneys and warm or invigorate yang

Kidney vacuity with water spilling over: Supplement the kidneys, warm yang, and seep water

Kidney yin vacuity: Supplement the kidneys and enrich or nourish yin

Yin vacuity-fire effulgence: Supplement the kidneys, enrich yin, and drain fire

Kidney essence insufficiency: Supplement the kidneys and fill, foster, or boost the essence

Urinary bladder damp heat: Clear heat, disinhibit dampness, and free the flow of strangury

APPENDIX III

Patient Herb Instruction Form

Because most Western patients are not experienced taking Chinese herbal medicinals, it is important to provide them with clear, simple, written instructions on how to take their Chinese herbal medications. For pills and powders, this is easy and straightforward. For decocted Chinese medicinals, this can be a bit more complicated. However, even if one prescribes bulk-dispensed decocted formulas, one can design a preprinted form that can be quickly and easily personalized for each patient. Below is a sample of one such form.

Sample Herbal Instruction Form

Pills (tablets, capsules):

1. _____ (pill name or identifier)
Take ____ pills each time, _____ times per day (before) (after) (with) meals.
2. _____ (pill name or identifier)
Take ____ pills each time, _____ times per day (before) (after) (with) meals.
3. _____ (pill name or identifier)
Take ____ pills each time, _____ times per day (before) (after) (with) meals.

Powders:

_____ (powder name or identifier)
Take _____ spoonfuls (of the spoon provided), _____ times per day (before) (after) (with meals.)
_____ (powder name or identifier)
Take _____ spoonfuls (of the spoon provided), _____ times per day (before) (after) (with meals.)
_____ (powder name or identifier)
Take _____ spoonfuls (of the spoon provided), _____ times per day (before) (after) (with meals.)

Decoctions:

[Depending on how you have been taught to prescribe Chinese herbs in decoction, you will want to create a similar form for your patients to the one below. Such a form will provide your patients with clear, unambiguous directions for how to prepare their Chinese herbal decoctions. This will save you time with oral instructions and help prevent any legal problems due to imprecise or faulty instructions. What you decide to include on this form is entirely up to you and can be modified for the exigencies of your clinic.]

To get the most effect out of your Chinese herbal prescription, please follow the checked instructions on this sheet. If you have any questions about any of these instructions, please do not hesitate to ask for help at the front desk or call between the hours of _____ to _____, Monday-Friday.

Please use a lidded glass, ceramic, or enameled pot to cook your Chinese herbs. Please do not use iron, steel, aluminum, or copper pots.

You have been given ___ packets of herbs which are meant to last you ____ days.

__ Cook any herbs in a separate packet marked "Precook herbs" for 45 minutes in _____ Cups of water at a medium boil in a covered pot. At the end of this time, add more water to replace what has been boiled away.

__ If there are no pre-cooked herbs, add the herbs in the packet marked "Main herbs" to ____ Cups of water and allow to soak for 20 minutes.

__ If there are pre-cooked herbs, add the herbs in the packet marked "Main herbs" to the pre-cooked herbs and cook for another _____ minutes at a _____ boil.

__ If there are any herbs in a packet marked "Add later," add these herbs at the end of cooking the main herbs. Turn the heat down to simmer and cook for 5-7 minutes maximum.

__ If there are any herbs in a packet marked "Steep," add these herbs after turning off the heat completely and allow to steep for 7-10 minutes.

__ If there are any herbs in a packet marked "Dissolve," first strain the cooked herbs and reserve the medicinal liquid. While still hot, add these herbs to the hot decoction and stir till dissolved.

__ If the final liquid makes less than ____ Cups, add enough water to bring it up to that amount.

__ Take ____ Cups of medicinal liquid ____ per day 15-20 minutes _____ meals.

Take __ room temperature ____ warm.

__ You may save the dregs from two days batches, combine, and recook for a third day's dose. In that case, please add any fresh "Add later," "Steep," or "Dissolve" herbs as described above. These extra herbs have been included in your prescription.

If the medicinal liquid is very bad tasting, you may suck on a couple of raisons or small piece of dried fruit to help clear your palate. However, do not add sugar, honey, or any other flavoring unless specifically instructed to do so. Although this flavor should not change, if the herbs are correct for your condition, your negative reaction to them should change after only a couple-few days.

Some Chinese doctors believe that the medicinal effects of the herbs begin with the inhalation of the smell of the cooking herbs.

You may store the medicinal liquid in the refrigerator for 2-3 days. However, if the liquid changes taste, please discard and start a new batch.

This formula is based on your signs and symptoms on the day it was prescribed. If you happen to catch cold or develop new symptoms, please call your practitioner before taking or continuing to take this formula.

___ The last day of this current prescription, please call your practitioner in order to discuss your current signs and symptoms so that a new prescription can be written and filled for you.

APPENDIX IV

Problem Based Learning Exercise Answers

Chapter 2

1. Stomach heat: Large or normal appetite, possible bad breath, possible yellow tongue fur; spleen vacuity: fatigue, orthostatic hypotension, easy bleeding, loose stools; spleen vacuity with dampness: a fat, enlarged tongue with teeth-marks on its edges, slimy tongue fur. Pulse signs: a soggy, possibly also slippery pulse in the right bar position.

2.

A. Low-grade and/or tidal fever, heat in the five centers, hot flashes, malar flushing, a red tongue with scanty fur, and a fine, rapid or surging, rapid pulse

B. Fatigue, a pale or sallow yellow facial complexion, heart palpitations, pale lips and nails, brittle nails, a pale tongue with thin, white fur, and a fine, forceless pulse

C. Acute onset of disease which has persisted for several days, alternating fever and chills, lack of appetite, possible nausea, a tongue with a combination of white and yellow fur, and a bowstring, rapid pulse

D. Chronic, persistent vaginal discharge with possible external genital itching and/or burning, possible frequent, urgent, and/or painful urination, possible red, pustular

skin lesions or skin lesions associated with prominent
swelling or seepage, possible chronic burning, loose stools
which are bright yellow in color and accompanied by a
foul odor, fatigue, lack of strength, heart palpitations,
insomnia, a pale or sallow yellow facial complexion but
flushed cheeks in the afternoon, heat in the five centers, a
fat, teeth-marked tongue which is pale in color but has a
bright red tip and scanty, slimy, yellow fur, and a fine,
rapid or soggy, rapid pulse in the inch and/or bar positions
but deep, fine, and slippery in the cubit positions

3. A bowstring, slow pulse suggests liver depression qi stagnation or at least some blockage and obstruction plus yang
vacuity. To determine if there is liver depression, one should
ask if the patient is at all irritable. To determine if there is
yang vacuity, ask if there are cold feet, nocturia, low back
soreness and weakness, aversion of cold, a predilection for
warm drinks, and decreased libido.

The two basic mechanisms for a slow pulse are A) not enough
yang qi to stir the pulse at its proper speed or B) some evil qi
blocking and hindering the free flow of the qi and blood.

4.
A. Hot, dry stomach: Rapid hungering, yellow tongue fur
(heat), thirst or a dry mouth and throat, chapped lips, dry
tongue fur (dryness)
B. Vacuous, cold, damp spleen: Fatigue, cold hands and
feet, orthostatic hypotension, lack of strength, a fat
tongue with teeth-marks on its edges
C. Diarrhea with light yellow stools, possible foul odor,
possible anal itching or burning with defecation, possible
explosive stools
D. Low back soreness and weakness, nocturia, clear, long
urination, decreased libido

The bar position pulse on the right might be soggy if spleen vacuity and dampness are more prominent or floating and slippery if stomach heat is more prominent. The cubit positions will typically be deep, bowstring, and slippery. If heat and cold are reasonably equal, the pulse will be normal in speed, one cancelling out the other's pulse sign in terms of rate.

If spleen vacuity and dampness are at the heart of this problem, then one should chose a guiding formula from the qi-supplementing category which also seeps and eliminates dampness. *Shen Ling Bai Zhu San* (Ginseng, Poria & Atractylodes Powder) is one such formula. It should then be modified to clear and eliminate dampness and heat from the intestines by the addition of bitter, cold medicinals, such as *Huang Qin* (Radix Scutellariae Baicalensis), *Huang Lian* (Rhizoma Coptidis Chinensis), and/or *Huang Bai* (Cortex Phellodendri).

5. Tinnitus, dizziness, low back soreness and pain, matitudinal insomnia, nocturia but scanty, yellow urine

6. For low back pain associated with yin vacuity, one might add *Sang Ji Sheng* (Ramulus Loranthi Seu Visci), *Gou Qi Zi* (Fructus Lycii Chinensis), and *Du Zhong* (Cortex Eucommiae Ulmoidis). For night sweats, one might add *Fu Xiao Mai* (Fructus Levis Tritici Aestivi) and *Mu Li* (Concha Ostreae).

7. Loose stools, edema, heavy, distended headache, bodily heaviness and encumbrance, possible leukorrhea in a female, possible pale-colored, swollen skin lesions

Case history exercises

Case 1

1. Heat, qi vacuity, and blood stasis
2. Yin reaches its extreme and transforms into yang
3. Yin vacuity/vacuity heat

4. The small secondary sexual characteristics, premature grey hair, late menarche, low back pain, frequent, darkish, but scanty urination, and nocturia all point to kidney yin vacuity. The night sweats, red facial complexion, agitation, red tongue, and fine, rapid pulse all point to vacuity heat.

5. Former heaven natural endowment yin insufficiency

6. All damage and consume yin fluids

7. To supplement the kidneys and enrich yin, clear heat and stop bleeding

8. Treatment should commence immediately at the end of menstruation.

9. *Zhi Bai Di Huang Wan Jia Wei* (Anemarrhena & Phellodendron Rehmannia Pills with Added Flavors)

Zhi Mu (Rhizoma Anemarrhenae Aspheloidis), 9 parts
Huang Bai (Cortex Phellodendri), 9 parts
Shu Di (cooked Radix Rehmanniae Glutinosae), 9 parts
Sheng Di (uncooked Radix Rehmanniae Glutinosae), 15 parts
Han Lian Cao (Herba Ecliptae Prostratae), 15 parts
Nu Zhen Zi (Fructus Ligustri Lucidi), 15 parts
Mu Dan Pi (Cortex Radicis Moutan), 9 parts
Shan Zhu Yu (Fructus Corni Officinalis), 9 parts
Shan Yao (Radix Dioscoreae Oppositae), 9 parts
Fu Ling (Sclerotium Poriae Cocos), 9 parts
Ze Xie (Rhizoma Alismatis Orientalis), 9 parts

Case 2

1. Insufficient qi to expel the urine or some evil qi blocking and hindering the expulsion of urine

2. Symptoms associated with both kidney vacuity and blood stasis are commonly worse at night.

3. Benign prostatic hypertrophy (BPH)

4. Get a digital rectal exam (DRE) and a prostate specific antigen (PSA) blood test to rule out prostate cancer

5. Spleen-kidney dual vacuity with probable blood stasis

6. BPH is a chronic condition associated with age. In addi-

tion, both qi vacuity and yang vacuity may lead to blood stasis. Therefore, this saying suggests the likelihood of blood stasis complicating this man's condition.

7. Fortify the spleen and boost the qi, supplement the kidneys and invigorate yang, quicken the blood and free the flow of the network vessels, secure the essence

8. Probably this man should be prescribed Chinese herbs in the form of an extract powder due to two facts: A) he will need medication over a prolonged period of time, *i.e.*, months and years, and B) he will probably need, at least at first, an individually written prescription. Later on, he might be able to be switched to a ready-made pill or capsule, but it is probable that, at the beginning, he will need a personally written formula.

9. *Bu Zhong Yi Qi Tang He Jin Suo Gu Jing Wan Jia Jian* (Supplement the Center & Boost the Qi Decoction Plus Golden Lock Secure the Essence Pills with Additions & Subtractions)

Huang Qi (Radix Astragali Membranacei), 18 parts
Dang Shen (Radix Codonopsitis Pilosulae), 9 parts
Bai Zhu (Rhizoma Atractylodis Macrocephalae), 9 parts
Fu Ling (Sclerotium Poriae Cocos), 12 parts
Qian Shi (Semen Euryalis Fercois), 9 parts
Sha Yuan Zi (Semen Astragali Complanati), 15 parts
Lian Zi (Semen Nelumbinis Nuciferae), 9 parts
Dang Gui (Radix Angelicae Sinensis), 9 parts
Niu Xi (Radix Achyranthis Bidentatae), 9 parts
Chen Pi (Pericarpium Citri Reticulatae), 6 parts
mix-fried *Gan Cao* (Radix Glycyrrhizae Uralensis), 6 parts
Sheng Ma (Rhizoma Cimicifugae), 6 parts
Chai Hu (Radix Bupleuri), 3 parts
Di Long (Lumbricus), 3 parts

Case 3

1. Taxation strangury (*lao lin*)
2. Liver-spleen disharmony with blood stasis

3. Irritability, premenstrual breast distention and pain, and bowstring pulse indicate liver depression qi stagnation. Fatigue, loose stools, craving for sweets, sagging feeling in the lower abdomen, orthostatic hypotension, hemorrhoids when standing, and a fat tongue with teethmarks on its edges indicate spleen qi vacuity. Dyspareunia indicates blood stasis.

4. Downward falling of the central qi

5. Dyspareunia means poking pain with intercourse. It's a hallaleulia symptom indicating blood stasis.

6. If there is pain, there is no free flow.

7. Fortify the spleen and boost the qi, course the liver and dis-inhibit the qi mechanism, lift the fallen and quicken the blood

8. To achieve speedy results in a short period of time, this woman should first be treated with bulk-dispensed herbs in a water-based decoction. Then, to secure and stabilize the therapeutic effects, she should be treated with either ready-made pills or extract powders at a low dose but for some time.

9. *Bu Zhong Yi Qi Tang Jia Wei* (Supplement the Center & Boost the Qi Decoction with Added Flavors)

Huang Qi (Radix Astragali Membranacei), 18 parts
Dang Shen (Radix Codonopsitis Pilosulae), 9 parts
Bai Zhu (Rhizoma Atractylodis Macrocephalae), 9 parts
Fu Ling (Sclerotium Poriae Cocos), 12 parts
Dang Gui (Radix Angelicae Sinensis), 9 parts
Bai Shao (Radix Albus Paeoniae Lactiflorae), 9 parts
Zhi Ke (Fructus Citri Aurantii), 6 parts
Chen Pi (Pericarpium Citri Reticulatae), 6 parts
mix-fried *Gan Cao* (Radix Glycyrrhizae Uralensis), 6 parts
Sheng Ma (Rhizoma Cimicifugae), 6 parts
Chai Hu (Radix Bupleuri), 9 parts

Case 4

1. To physically describe the skin lesions in terms of shape, size, color, location, and type

2. Hand and foot yang ming

3. Liver depression transforming depressive heat which has mutually engendered heat in the stomach and intestines combined with some dampness and turbidity. This depressive heat is then floating upward to steam the lungs.

4. Irritability, premenstrual breast distention and pain, lower abdominal bloating, the dark, dusky colored tongue, and a bowstring pulse indicate liver depression. Bad breath, bleeding gums, the acne along the course of the yang ming, the constipation, the dry, yellow tongue fur, and the surging, rapid pulse indicate heat in the stomach and intestines.

5. No

6. As stated above in answer #3

7. Course the liver and resolve depression, clear heat from the lungs, liver, stomach, and intestines, eliminate dampness and transform turbidity

8. *Xiao Chai Hu Tang Jia Jian* (Minor Bupleurum Decoction with Additions & Subtractions)

Chai Hu (Radix Bupleuri), 9 parts
Huang Qin (Radix Scutellariae Baicalensis), 12 parts
Pi Ba Ye (Folium Eriobotryae Japonicae), 9 parts
Ban Xia (Rhizoma Pinelliae Ternatae), 9 parts
Dang Gui (Radix Angelicae Sinensis), 9 parts
Bai Shao (Radix Albus Paeoniae Lactiflorae), 9 parts
Xiang Fu (Rhizoma Cyperi Rotundi), 9 parts
Sheng Jiang (uncooked Rhizoma Zingiberis Officinalis), 6 parts
Da Zao (Fructus Zizyphi Jujubae), 6 parts
mix-fried *Gan Cao* (Radix Glycyrrhizae Uralensis), 4.5 parts

9. The patient should be advised not to drink alcohol or to eat greasy, fried, spicy, or hot-flavored foods.

Case 5

1. Wind damp heat impediment pain

2. Liver-spleen disharmony

3. The fatigue, loose stools, and the fat tongue with teeth-marks on it edges indicate spleen vacuity. The irritability and bowstring pulse indicate liver depression.

4. Harmonize the liver and spleen, clear heat and eliminate dampness, free the flow of impediment and stop pain

5. *Dang Gui Nian Tong Tang* (Dang Gui Assuage Pain Decoction)

Dang Gui (Radix Angelicae Sinensis), 12g
Dang Shen (Radix Codonopsitis Pilosulae), 9g
Bai Zhu (Rhizoma Atractylodis Macrocephalae), 9g
Cang Zhu (Rhizoma Atractylodis), 9g
Zhu Ling (Sclerotium Polypori Umbellati), 12g
Ze Xie (Rhizoma Alismatis Orientalis), 9g
Huang Qin (Radix Scutellariae Baicalensis), 9g
Yin Chen Hao (Herba Artemisiae Capillaris), 9g
Ku Shen (Radix Sophorae Flavescentis), 9g
Ge Gen (Radix Puerariae Lobatae), 9g
Qiang Huo (Radix Et Rhizoma Notopterygii), 9g
Fang Feng (Radix Ledebouriellae Divaricatae), 9g
Sheng Ma (Rhizoma Cimicifugae), 6g
Gan Cao (Radix Glycyrrhizae Uralensis), 3g

6. Stay away from sugar and sweets, fried, fatty, greasy foods, hot, spicy, peppery foods, alcohol, and too many dairy products.

7. Due to a liver-spleen disharmony, there is spleen vacuity failing to control the movement and transformation of water fluids. These collect and transform into damp evils. Damp evils are heavy and turbid and tend to seep downward. This is especially the case premenstrually when A) the liver typically becomes more depressed if deprived from sufficient blood to nourish it adequately and B) when the heart qi sends both blood and fluids downward to accumulate in the uterus. Because fluids are thinner than blood, they arrive first. If these fluids then block the

free flow of yang qi in the lower burner, they may give rise to depressive heat. If this depressive heat combines with the damp evils, this transforms into damp heat.

Case 6

1. Spleen qi vacuity
2. Food stagnation transforming heat
3. Stomach heat
4. Spleen qi vacuity with stomach heat and food stagnation. In all probability, there is also liver depression based on the saying that, in infants, the liver commonly has a surplus, and both spleen vacuity and food stagnation may lead to liver depression.
5. Fortify the spleen and supplement the qi, clear the stomach and abduct stagnation, free the flow of the stools and stop pain
6. The earache and the constipation
7. *Xiao Chai Hu Tang Jia Wei* (Minor Bupleurum Decoction with Added Flavors)

Chai Hu (Radix Bupleuri), 9 parts
Huang Qin (Radix Scutellariae Baicalensis), 12 parts
Lian Qiao (Fructus Forsythiae Suspensae), 9 parts
Jin Yin Hua (Flos Lonicerae Japonicae), 9 parts
Ban Xia (Rhizoma Pinelliae Ternatae), 9 parts
Chuan Xiong (Radix Ligustici Wallichii), 15 parts
Bai Zhi (Radix Angelicae Dahuricae), 9 parts
Shi Chang Pu (Rhizoma Acori Graminei), 9parts
Shan Zha (Fructus Crataegi), 9parts
Ji Nei Jin (Endothelium Gigeriae Galli), 9parts
Sheng Jiang (uncooked Rhizoma Zingiberis Officinalis),
        6 parts
Da Zao (Fructus Zizyphi Jujubae), 6 parts
mix-fried *Gan Cao* (Radix Glycyrrhizae Uralensis), 6 parts

8. It can either be made into an extract powder and dissolved in water or it may be made as a decoction. In

either case, the liquid will be administered by eye-dropper, paying more attention to small, frequent administrations that the total dose per day.

Chapter 3

1. First aid in emergency conditions. These ready-made medicines could be stored long-term against use and could simply be mixed with water in order to administer. Therefore, they were readily at hand and quickly administered.

2. At low doses, extract powders are probably more cost effective for patients. However, once the dose goes over a certain amount, extract powders become prohibitively expensive and bulk-dispensed, water-based decoctions typically become more economical. This depends, of course, on the wholesale price a practitioner can get for each of these types of medicinals.

3. Increase. This is because remedial treatment of active disease usually requires larger doses. Ready-made pills are not really made for the remedial treatment of active disease. They are more for preventive therapy and regulating and rectifying treatment after the symptoms of active disease have largely been eliminated or at least stabilized.

4. No, all powdered extracts are not equally potent. This is because different manufacturers make their powders to different concentration ratios. While most are 5:1 extracts, some are 7:1, and others may go as high as 15:1 for a formula and 20:1 for a single medicinal.

5. Powders may either be extracts or simply ground up crude herbs. Extracts are more potent then simple herb powders because they are concentrates.

6. The drawback is that they are not capable of being modified once they are made up, whereas bulk-dispensed medicinals administered as a water-based decoction can be exactly modified for a patient's personal needs day by day if necessary.

7. The cost-benefit ratio helps one determine if the cost of a therapy, in terms of money, time, and/or trouble, is worth the anticipated benefit. For instance, a large formula administered as a water-based decoction may be worth the cost in time and money for a patient suffering from a severe, acute migraine headache. However, for a patient simply trying to prevent a headache that has not occurred and may not occur, such a water-based decoction may not be worth the time and money. In that case, a cheaper, easier-to-take form of Chinese medicine which can be taken day after day for weeks on end may be better.

8. In pill form because pills are so easy to store and take. If the patient stops taking a more time-consuming, distasteful, or expensive form of medication prematurely, this is not so good. Therefore, ease of storage and administration definitely affects patient adherence to the therapeutic regime.

Chapter 4

1. One would have to give 30 grams of a 5:1 extract and 21 grams of a 7:1 extract to equal the equivalent of 150 grams in decoction.

2. 2.5 grams

3. Since six grams of a 5:1 extract only equals 30 grams in decoction, you should increase the number of grams per day in order to come closer to the 200 grams per day that have been proven to be effective. Doubling the dose to 12 grams per day would equal 60 grams in decoction, while quadrupling it to 24 grams would equal 120 grams in decoction.

While this is still substantially less than 200 grams per day, it should achieve a better effect than the manufacturer's standard recommendation.

4. When a practitioner prescribes a standardized extract fraction of an herb based on the assumption that the chemical in question is the therapeutically active ingredient, this assumption may or may not be true. The chemical may not be, in fact, the active ingredient. In that case, there would be no therapeutic effect. It may also be possible that the chemical is the *main* active ingredient, but, in order for it to get its effect, it must be taken along with some other cofactor or cofactors. If that cofactor is not present, the chemical may still not get its intended effect. Further, it is possible that other chemical constituents of a whole herbal medicinal may buffer or negate any unwanted side effects that the single ingredient would otherwise cause. And finally, it is possible that an herbal medicinal may contain a main active ingredient but several other similar but less potent active ingredients. In such a case, one may need to use less of the whole herbal medicinal to achieve the same intended effect, since the other ingredients are also working towards the same effect. Since many side effects are dose-dependent, using this smaller dose of the main active ingredient along with its similar ingredients in the whole medicinal may achieve the intended effect without provoking any side effects.

Chapter 5

1. 2/5 the adult dosage = 60 grams

2. 167% of the adult dosage = 10 grams

3.

A. Acute condition
B. If taken as a bulk-dispensed, water-based decoction with only the standard ingredients, the daily dose would be

between 24-48 grams per day depending on the size and age of the patient and the severity of the condition.

4. One way to determine the optimal dose to prevent regression would be to prescribe the equivalent of 75% of the previous daily decoction they were treated remedially with. After two weeks, the patient's blood glucose could be checked to see if there was any change. If the blood glucose had gone back up, the dosage would need to be increased. If the blood glucose had remained steady, the dose might be decreased to 50% of the previous daily decoction. After another two weeks, if the blood sugar had gone up, one would know that the right dosage was somewhere between 50-75% of the decoction. If the blood glucose was still normal, one could reduce the dosage to 25% and see what happened to the blood glucose, adjusting the dosage up or down accordingly.

Another correct answer to this question would be to determine whether the qi or the yin vacuity was more prominent based on the number and severity of the signs and symptoms of each. If one pattern was more prominent than the other, one would give more of the one formula and less of the other. If both patterns were equally prominent, then one would give the same amount of both formulas.

In fact, these two answers supplement each other.

5. 40 grams

6. The patient has an acute condition which is quite painful. That suggests he should be treated with the quickest-acting, strongest Chinese medicine possible. In that case, that means taking a water-based decoction. Since this form of administration should achieve its intended effect in a matter of hours or at most a day, the patient will not have to make and take such decoctions long-term—only a couple-few days at most. You might end by asking the patient if he wants to see his pain disappear as quickly as possible. If he answers yes, then say that taking the decoction is the way to make that happen. In addition, you might close by saying that it is what I certainly would do for myself if I were in such discomfort.

7.
  A. 3-6g
  B. 9-30g
  C. 6-15g
  D. 3-9g
  E. 3-9g
  F. 9-15g
  G. 6-9g
  H. 3-9g
  I. 9-15g
  J. 6-15g
  K. 9-15g
  L. 3-9g
  M. 6-12g
  N. 4.5-15g
  O. 9-30g
  P. 9-15g

8. A low trial dose because she is more sensitive than normal. The standard daily dose is likely to cause unwanted side effects. If the low trial dose does not cause any adverse reactions, one can always increase the dose.

9. Depending on the schedule of acupuncture, it should decrease the required dose of Chinese herbal medicinals. This is because one is treating with two separate modalities. In the Chinese medical literature, standard daily doses are based on the patient's only being treated by a single modality, *i.e.,* internally administered herbal medicinals. However, if now one is treating with two modalities, this should achieve the desired therapeutic effect with a lesser dose of the Chinese medicinals. That is, as long as the acupuncture treatment is given often enough to have a real impact on the patient's condition.

10. Because the patient's condition is more serious, in fact, life-threatening, you want to improve this patient's condition as quickly as possible. Therefore, the higher dose makes sense.

11. Because the patient's condition is less severe than the one with active RA. In this case, one is simply trying to keep the patient in remission as long and as completely as possible. As long as the patient follows his or her practitioner's advice in terms of diet and lifestyle, a smaller dose of Chinese medicinals should be all that is necessary to accomplish those goals. Since the patient is going to have to take these Chinese herbs for a prolonged, indefinite period of time, the practitioner also should make their administration as quick and easy as possible so as to foster adherence.

12. Again, the patient with kidney failure is suffering from a life-threatening condition, while the patient with interstitial cystitis is simply suffering from a nagging discomfort. This means that the patient with kidney failure needs to be treated as quickly as possible. The patient with interstitial cystitis, on the other hand, can be treated with an easier, more relaxed protocol involving not only lower doses but an easier mode of administration.

Chapter 6

1. Assume that the patient has changed something about his diet and/or lifestyle.

2. Have you changed your diet? If so, how? Have you changed your lifestyle? If so, how? Are you under more stress lately? If so, in what way? Are you exercising more/less? If so, how/why? Have you changed anything about the way you are taking your herbs? If so, how/what? Do the herbs taste the same as always? If not, how has their taste changed?

3. The patient's pattern(s) has/have changed enough that the medicinals are not correct.

4. Redo his or her pattern discrimination by asking about current symptoms, looking at the patient's tongue, and feeling the patient's pulse.

5. Have the patient take a few days of the medicinals to see if the problem is merely one of habituation. If that turns out not to be the problem, then the next thing to try is upping the patient's dose.

Chapter 7

There's no way to provide answers to these questions. They are dependent on what the reader finds out when they do their on-line search and when they contact their supplier(s).

Chapter 8

Some potentially fetotoxic Chinese medicinals include:

Qian Niu Zi (Semen Pharbiditis)
Gan Sui (Radix Euphorbiae Kansui)
Yuan Hua (Flos Daphhis Genkwae)
Jing Da Ji (Radix Euphrobiae Seu Knoxiae)
Shang Lu (Radix Phytolaccae)
Tian Hua Fen (Radix Trichosanthis Kirlowii)
Bai Fu Zi (Rhizoma Typhonii Gigantei Seu Radix Aconiti Koreani)
Zao Jiao (Fructus Gleditschiae Chinensis)
Zao Jiao Ci (Spina Gleditschiae Chinensis)
Fu Zi (Radix Lateralis Praeparatus Aconiti Carmichaeli)
Wu Gong (Scolopendra Subspinipes)
Qing Fen (Calomelas)
Xiong Huang (Realgar)
Liu Huang (Sulphur)
Ma Qian Zi (Semen Strychnotis Nuxvomicae)
Mu Bie Zi (Semen Mormordicae Cochinensis)
Zhang Nao (Camphora)

Ban Mao (Mylabris)
Chan Su (Secretio Bufonis)
Kuan Jin Teng (Caulis Tinosporae Sinensis)

1.Nephrotoxicity, hepatotoxicity, and fetotoxicity

2. Aristolochic acid (AA)

3. *Guang Fang Ji* (Radix Aristolochiae Fangji) or *Xi Xin* (Herba Asari Cum Radice)

4.
   A. Isoniazid
   B. Tetracyclines
   C. Rifampcin
   D. Chlorpromazine
   E. Erythromycin

5.
   A. Previous notable adverse reactions to drugs or herbs
   B. A history of a number of different allergies
   C. A history of chronic skin rashes
   D. Pre-existing liver disease

6.
   A. Skin rash
   B. Nausea or bloating
   C. Worsening fatigue
   D. Aching in the area of the liver, jaundice, reduction in the color of the feces

7.
   Qian Niu Zi (Semen Pharbiditis)
   Gan Sui (Radix Euphorbiae Kansui)
   Shang Lu (Radix Phytolaccae)
   Tian Hua Fen (Radix Trichosanthis Kirlowii)
   Bai Fu Zi (Rhizoma Typhonii Gigantei Seu Radix Aconiti
       Koreani)

Zao Jiao (Fructus Gleditschiae Chinensis)
Zao Jiao Ci (Spina Gleditschiae Chinensis)
Fu Zi (Radix Lateralis Praeparatus Aconiti Carmichaeli)
Wu Gong (Scolopendra Subspinipes)
Qing Fen (Calomelas)
Xiong Huang (Realgar)
Liu Huang (Sulphur)
Ma Qian Zi (Semen Strychnotis)

8. Blood-quickeners

Chapter 9

Case history exercises

Case 1

1. Heat, qi vacuity, and blood stasis
2. Restless stirring of the fetus or fetal stirring & restlessness
3. Qi vacuity, liver depression, and blood stasis
4. Fatigue, forceless pulse, pinkish, dilute blood, and fat tongue = qi vacuity
PMS, bowstring pulse = liver depression
Painful menstruation, sooty complexion, and fixed lower abdominal pain = blood stasis
5. Fortify the spleen and boost the qi, course the liver and rectify the qi, quicken the blood and quiet the fetus
6. *Tian Qi* (Radix Pseudoginseng), *Yi Mu Cao* (Herba Leonuri Heterophylli)
7. Yes
8. N/A
9. Just until the bleeding stops

Case 2

1. Nausea & vomiting during pregnancy
2. Yin vacuity with upward counterflow of the stomach qi

3. Enrich yin and engender fluids, harmonize the stomach and stop vomiting

4. *Mai Men Dong* because 1) it enriches yin and engenders fluids in the stomach, and 2) *Tian Hua Fen* is an abortifacient and *Mai Men Dong* is not

5. *Mai Men Dong Tang* (Ophiopogon Decoction) from the *Jin Gui Yao Lue* (Essentials from the *Golden Cabinet*)

   Mai Men Dong (Tuber Ophiopogonis Japonici), 12g

   Ban Xia (Rhizoma Pinelliae Ternatae), 9g

   Gu Ya (Fructus Germinatus Oryzae Sativae), 9g

   Ren Shen (Radix Panacis Ginseng), 4.5g

   Da Zao (Fructus Zizyphi Jujubae), 5 pieces

   mix-fried *Gan Cao* (Radix Glycyrrhizae Uralensis), 3-6g

6. In decoction because the liquid will be easier to absorb

7. Sip by sip at frequent intervals

8. Rubbing some fresh ginger on her tongue and under her nose before drinking the decoction

9. She can take her decocted herbs either warm or room temperature. On the one hand, warm decoctions are better for supplementation. On the other, there is some vacuity heat. So taking the decoction at room temperature is also OK.

Case 3

1. Heat toxins and blood dryness

2. Clear heat and resolve toxins, nourish the blood and moisten dryness

3. Probably not. Psoriasis is a very deep-seated and recalcitrant condition.

4. Typically, toxin-resolving, cancer-combating medicinals are used in the treatment of psoriasis internally. Some of these may themselves be toxic based on the saying, "Combat toxins with toxins."

5. Heat toxins, in the form of fetal toxins, are believed to be transferable from the mother to the child. However, this

transfer occurs during gestation, not breast-feeding. Medicinals which clear heat from the blood aspect or division and resolve toxins include:

Zi Cao (Radix Lithospermi Seu Arnebiae)
Ban Lan Gen (Radix Isatidis Seu Baphicanthi)
Dan Pi (Cortex Radicis Moutan)
Sheng Di (uncooked Radix Rehmanniae Glutinosae)
Pu Gong Ying (Herba Taraxaci Mongolici Cum Radice)

6. *Pu Gong Ying* not only clears heat and resolves toxins, it also frees the flow of the breasts and increases milk production. In addition, because the breast milk is manufactured out of the blood, nourishing the blood and moistening dryness will also increase the quantity and quality of the breast milk.

7. No

Chapter 10

1. Harmonizing the liver and spleen means to course the liver and rectify the qi at the same time as fortifying the spleen and supplementing or boosting the qi.

2. Harmonizing the liver and stomach means to course the liver and rectify the qi at the same time as harmonizing the stomach and downbearing counterflow.

3. Harmonizing the spleen and stomach means to fortify the spleen and supplement or boost the qi at the same time as harmonizing the stomach and downbearing counterflow.

4. Harmonizing the stomach and intestines means to clear heat from the stomach and intestines at the same time as downbearing upward counterflow of the stomach and stopping intestinal diarrhea.

5. It means to resolve depression by upbearing and pushing outward the yang qi.

6. Because acrid, exterior-resolving medicinals upbear and out-thrust the yang qi.

7. Harmonize the liver and spleen, drain the stomach and clear heat, transform phlegm and scatter nodulation or binding, and quicken the blood and transform stasis

> *Xiao Chai Hu Tang Jia Wei* (Minor Bupleurum Decoction with Added Flavors)
> *Chai Hu* (Radix Bupleuri), 9g
> *Huang Qin* (Radix Scutellariae Baicalensis), 12g
> *Ban Xia* (Rhizoma Pinelliae Ternatae), 9g
> *Dang Shen* (Radix Codonopsitis Pilosulae), 9g
> *Dan Pi* (Cortex Radicis Moutan), 9g
> *Chi Shao* (Radix Rubrus Paeoniae Lactiflorae), 9g
> *Dang Gui* (Radix Angelicae Sinensis), 9g
> *Hai Zao* (Herba Sargassii), 9g
> *Mu Li* (Concha Ostreae), 12g
> *Xia Ku Cao* (Spica Prunellae Vulgaris), 15g
> mix-fried *Gan Cao* (Radix Glycyrrhizae Uralensis), 6g
> *Sheng Jiang* (uncooked Rhizoma Zingiberis Officinalis), 2 slices
> *Da Zao* (Fructus Zizyphi Jujubae), 3 pieces

8. Harmonize the liver and spleen, nourish the blood, clear the stomach, and abduct stagnation

Xiao Chai Hu Tang Jia Wei (Minor Bupleurum Decoction with Added Flavors)
> *Chai Hu* (Radix Bupleuri), 9g
> *Huang Qin* (Radix Scutellariae Baicalensis), 12g
> *Ban Xia* (Rhizoma Pinelliae Ternatae), 9g
> *Dang Shen* (Radix Codonopsitis Pilosulae), 9g
> *Xiang Fu* (Rhizoma Cyperi Rotundi), 9g
> *Dang Gui* (Radix Angelicae Sinensis), 9g
> *Bai Shao* (Radix Albus Paeoniae Lactiflorae), 9g
> *Chen Pi* (Pericarpium Citri Reticulatae), 6g
> *Qing Pi* (Pericarpium Citri Reticulatae Viride), 6g

Shen Qu (Massa Medica Fermentata), 6g
mix-fried *Gan Cao* (Radix Glycyrrhizae Uralensis), 6g
Sheng Jiang (uncooked Rhizoma Zingiberis Officinalis), 2
    slices
Da Zao (Fructus Zizyphi Jujubae), 3 pieces

9. Harmonize the liver and spleen, clear and eliminate damp heat in the intestines, stop diarrhea and stop bleeding

Xiao Chai Hu Tang Jia Wei (Minor Bupleurum Decoction with
    Added Flavors)
    Chai Hu (Radix Bupleuri), 9g
    Huang Qin (Radix Scutellariae Baicalensis), 12g
    Ban Xia (Rhizoma Pinelliae Ternatae), 9g
    Dang Shen (Radix Codonopsitis Pilosulae), 9g
    Bai Tou Weng (Radix Pulsatillae Sinensis), 12g
    Qin Pi (Cortex Fraxini), 9g
    Sheng Di (uncooked Radix Rehmanniae Glutinosae), 12g
    Dan Pi (Cortex Radicis Moutan), 9g
    Fu Ling (Sclerotium Poriae Cocos), 12g
    Bai Zhu (Rhizoma Atractylodis Macrocephalae), 9g
    Huang Lian (Rhizoma Coptidis Chinensis), 6g
    mix-fried *Gan Cao* (Radix Glycyrrhizae Uralensis), 6g
    Sheng Jiang (uncooked Rhizoma Zingiberis Officinalis), 2
        slices
    Da Zao (Fructus Zizyphi Jujubae), 3 pieces

10. Fortify the spleen and boost the qi, enrich yin, resolve depression, and quicken the blood
Yi Guan Jian Jia Wei (One Link Decoction with Added Flavors)
    mix-fried *Huang Qi* (Radix Astragali Membranacei), 30-60g
    Sheng Di (uncooked Radix Rehmanniae Glutinosae), 15g
    Sha Shen (Radix Glehniae Littoralis), 12g
    Mai Men Dong (Tuber Ophiopogonis Japonici), 12g
    Dang Gui (Radix Angelicae Sinensis), 9g

Gou Qi Zi (Fructus Lycii Chinenis), 9g

Dan Pi (Cortex Radicis Moutan), 9g

Dan Shen (Radix Salviae Miltiorrhizae), 9g

Chuan Lian Zi (Fructus Meliae Toosendan), 6-9g

mix-fried *Gan Cao* (Radix Glycyrrhizae Uralensis), 6-9g

Chapter 11

These don't have answers. They are projects that the reader/student must do for him- or herself.

APPENDIX V

A Representative List of Pesticides and Heavy Metals Tested by Western Companies Producing Ready-made Herbal Medicines

Organophosphate Pesticides

1,2-Dibromochloropropane
Acephate
Azinphos (Guthion)
Carbophenothion
Chlorpyrifos (Dursban)
Co Ral (Coumaphos)
Coumaphos (Co Ral)
Cycloate (Roneet)
Cygon (Dimethoate)
Cymoxanil
Deltamethrin
Demeton S
Diazinon
Dibrom (Naled)
Dichlorvos
Dimethoate (Cygon)
Disulfoton
Dursban (Chlorpyrifos)
Dyfonate (Fonofos)
EPN
Ethion
Ethyl Parathion
Fenamiphos (Nemacur Phenamiphos)

Fenchlorfos
Fenitrothion
Fensulfothion
Fenthion
Fenvalerate (Sanmarton)
Fonofos (Dyfonate)
Guthion (Azinphos)
Hexazinone (Velpar)
Imidan (Phosmet)
Malathion
Me-Parathion
Merphos-B
Methamidophos (Monitor)
Methidathion
Miclobutanil (Rally)
Mocap
Monitor (Methamidophos)
Monocrotophos (Monocron)
Naled (Dibrom)
Nemacur (Fenamiphos, Phenamiphos)
Oxydemeton-methyl
Permethrin
Permethrin Phorate
Phenamiphos (Nemacur, Fenamiphos)
Propiconazole (Tilt)
Phorate
Phosalone (Rubitox)
Phosdrin
Phosmet (Imidan)
Phoxim
Pirimicarb
Pirimiphos-methyl
Rally (Miclobutanil)
Roneet (Cycloate)
Rubitox (Phosalone)
Sanmarton (Fenvalerate)
Sulprofos
TDE
Tetrachlorvinfos
Tilt (Propiconazole)

Tokuthion
Trichloronate
Velpar (Hexazinone)

Reporting Limit = .05 ppm

Chlorinated Pesticides

4, 4 DDE
4, 4 DDD
4, 4 DDT
Alachlor
Aldrin
Asana (Esfenvalerate)
BHC-A (Alpha-Hexachlorocyclohexane)
BHC-B (Beta-Hexachlorocyclohexane)
BHC-D (Delta-Hexachlorocyclohexane)
BHC-G (Lindane)
Captan
Chlordane
Chlorfenvinfos
Chlorpyrifos (Dursban)
Chlorpyrifos-methyl
Cypermethrin
Dicofol (Kelthane)
Dieldrin
Diethofencarb
Dursban (Chlorpyrifos)
Dylox (Trichlorfon)
Endosulfan Sulfate
Endosulfan I and II
Endrin Aldehyde
Endrin
Esfenvalerate (Asana)
Euparen M (Tolyfluanide)
Fenvalerate
Heptachlor Epoxide
Heptachlor

Hexachlorobenzene
Kelthane (Dicofol)
Mavrik (Tau-Fluvalinate)
Methoxychlor
Mirex
Miclobutanil (Rally)
Omite (Propargite)
Pentachloroaniline
Pestanal
Procymidone
Pyrethrum
Pyrimethanil
Quintozene
Rally (Miclobutanil)
Tau-Fluvalinate (Mavrik)
Tolyfluanide (Euparen M)
Tolylfluanid
Triadimenol
Trichlorfon (Dylox)
Vinclozolin

Reporting Limit = .05 ppm

Testing for Heavy Metals

Herb samples should be tested for five heavy metals: Arsenic, Cadmium, Chromium, Lead and Mercury. Listed below are the reporting limits below which it is considered that none of the element is detectable. Parts per million (ppm) represents the number of milligrams per kilogram (mg/kg) of the element found in the tested formula.

Reporting Limits

Arsenic - .07 ppm

Lead - .05 ppm

Cadmium - .05 ppm

Mercury - .05 ppm

Chromium - .05 ppm

ACUPOINT POCKET REFERENCE
by Bob Flaws
ISBN 0-936185-93-7
ISBN 978-0-936185-93-4

ACUPUNCTURE & IVF
by Lifang Liang
ISBN 0-891845-24-1
ISBN 978-0-891845-24-6

ACUPUNCTURE FOR STROKE REHABILITATION
Three Decades of Information from China
by Hoy Ping Yee Chan, *et al.*
ISBN 1-891845-35-7
ISBN 978-1-891845-35-2

ACUPUNCTURE PHYSICAL MEDICINE:
An Acupuncture Touchpoint Approach to the
Treatment of Chronic Pain, Fatigue, and Stress
Disorders
by Mark Seem
ISBN 1-891845-13-6
ISBN 978-1-891845-13-0

AGING & BLOOD STASIS:
A New Approach to TCM Geriatrics
by Yan De-xin
ISBN 0-936185-63-6
ISBN 978-0-936185-63-7

BETTER BREAST HEALTH NATURALLY
with CHINESE MEDICINE
by Honora Lee Wolfe & Bob Flaws
ISBN 0-936185-90-2
ISBN 978-0-936185-90-3

BIOMEDICINE: A TEXTBOOK FOR PRACTITIONERS
OF ACUPUNCTURE AND ORIENTAL MEDICINE
by Bruce H. Robinson, MD
ISBN 1-891845-38-1
ISBN 978-1-891845-38-3

THE BOOK OF JOOK: Chinese Medicinal Porridges
by Bob Flaws
ISBN 0-936185-60-6
ISBN 978-0-936185-60-0

CHANNEL DIVERGENCES Deeper Pathways of the
Web
by Miki Shima and Charles Chase
ISBN 1-891845-15-2
ISBN 978-1-891845-15-4

CHINESE MEDICAL OBSTETRICS
by Bob Flaws
ISBN 1-891845-30-6
ISBN 978-1-891845-30-7

CHINESE MEDICAL PALMISTRY:
Your Health in Your Hand
by Zong Xiao-fan & Gary Liscum
ISBN 0-936185-64-3
ISBN 978-0-936185-64-4

CHINESE MEDICAL PSYCHIATRY
A Textbook and Clinical Manual
by Bob Flaws and James Lake, MD
ISBN 1-845891-17-9
ISBN 978-1-845891-17-8

CHINESE MEDICINAL TEAS: Simple, Proven, Folk
Formulas for Common Diseases & Promoting Health
by Zong Xiao-fan & Gary Liscum
ISBN 0-936185-76-7
ISBN 978-0-936185-76-7

CHINESE MEDICINAL WINES & ELIXIRS
by Bob Flaws   Revised Edition
ISBN 0-936185-58-9
ISBN 978-0-936185-58-3

CHINESE MEDICINE & HEALTHY WEIGHT
MANAGEMENT
An Evidence-based Integrated Approach
by Juliette Aiyana, L. Ac.
ISBN 1-891845-44-6
ISBN 978-1-891845-44-4

CHINESE PEDIATRIC MASSAGE THERAPY: A
Parent's & Practitioner's Guide to the Prevention &
Treatment of Childhood Illness
by Fan Ya-li
ISBN 0-936185-54-6
ISBN 978-0-936185-54-5

CHINESE SELF-MASSAGE THERAPY:
The Easy Way to Health
by Fan Ya-li
ISBN 0-936185-74-0
ISBN 978-0-936185-74-3

THE CLASSIC OF DIFFICULTIES:
A Translation of the *Nan Jing*
translation by Bob Flaws
ISBN 1-891845-07-1
ISBN 978-1-891845-07-9

A CLINICIAN'S GUIDE TO USING GRANULE
EXTRACTS
by Eric Brand
ISBN 1-891845-51-9
ISBN 978-1-891845-51-2

A COMPENDIUM OF CHINESE MEDICAL
MENSTRUAL DISEASES
by Bob Flaws
ISBN 1-891845-31-4
ISBN 978-1-891845-31-4

CONCISE CHINESE MATERIA MEDICA
by Eric Brand and Nigel Wiseman
ISBN 0-912111-82-8
ISBN 978-0-912111-82-7

CONTEMPORARY GYNECOLOGY: An Integrated
Chinese-Western Approach
by Lifang Liang
ISBN 1-891845-50-0
ISBN 978-1-891845-50-5

CONTROLLING DIABETES NATURALLY WITH
CHINESE MEDICINE
by Lynn Kuchinski
ISBN 0-936185-06-3
ISBN 978-0-936185-06-2

CURING ARTHRITIS NATURALLY WITH
CHINESE MEDICINE
by Douglas Frank & Bob Flaws
ISBN 0-936185-87-2
ISBN 978-0-936185-87-3

CURING DEPRESSION NATURALLY WITH
CHINESE MEDICINE
by Rosa Schnyer & Bob Flaws
ISBN 0-936185-94-5
ISBN 978-0-936185-94-1

CURING FIBROMYALGIA NATURALLY WITH
CHINESE MEDICINE
by Bob Flaws
ISBN 1-891845-09-8
ISBN 978-1-891845-09-3

CURING HAY FEVER NATURALLY WITH
CHINESE MEDICINE
by Bob Flaws
ISBN 0-936185-91-0
ISBN 978-0-936185-91-0

CURING HEADACHES NATURALLY WITH
CHINESE MEDICINE
by Bob Flaws
ISBN 0-936185-95-3
ISBN 978-0-936185-95-8

CURING IBS NATURALLY WITH CHINESE
MEDICINE
by Jane Bean Oberski
ISBN 1-891845-11-X
ISBN 978-1-891845-11-6

CURING INSOMNIA NATURALLY WITH
CHINESE MEDICINE
by Bob Flaws
ISBN 0-936185-86-4
ISBN 978-0-936185-86-6

CURING PMS NATURALLY WITH CHINESE
MEDICINE
by Bob Flaws
ISBN 0-936185-85-6
ISBN 978-0-936185-85-9

DISEASES OF THE KIDNEY & BLADDER
by Hoy Ping Yee Chan, et al.
ISBN 1-891845-37-3
ISBN 978-1-891845-35-6

THE DIVINE FARMER'S MATERIA MEDICA
A Translation of the Shen Nong Ben Cao
translation by Yang Shouz-hong
ISBN 0-936185-96-1
ISBN 978-0-936185-96-5

DUI YAO: THE ART OF COMBINING
CHINESE HERBAL MEDICINALS
by Philippe Sionneau
ISBN 0-936185-81-3
ISBN 978-0-936185-81-1

ENDOMETRIOSIS, INFERTILITY AND
TRADITIONAL CHINESE MEDICINE:
A Layperson's Guide
by Bob Flaws
ISBN 0-936185-14-7
ISBN 978-0-936185-14-9

THE ESSENCE OF LIU FENG-WU'S GYNECOLOGY
by Liu Feng-wu, translated by Yang Shou-zhong
ISBN 0-936185-88-0
ISBN 978-0-936185-88-0

EXTRA TREATISES BASED ON INVESTIGATION &
INQUIRY: A Translation of Zhu Dan-xi's Ge Zhi Yu
Lun
translation by Yang Shou-zhong
ISBN 0-936185-53-8
ISBN 978-0-936185-53-8

FIRE IN THE VALLEY: TCM Diagnosis & Treatment of
Vaginal Diseases
by Bob Flaws
ISBN 0-936185-25-2
ISBN 978-0-936185-25-5

FULFILLING THE ESSENCE:
A Handbook of Traditional & Contemporary
Treatments for Female Infertility
by Bob Flaws
ISBN 0-936185-48-1
ISBN 978-0-936185-48-4

FU QING-ZHU'S GYNECOLOGY
trans. by Yang Shou-zhong and Liu Da-wei
ISBN 0-936185-35-X
ISBN 978-0-936185-35-4

GOLDEN NEEDLE WANG LE-TING: A 20th Century
Master's Approach to Acupuncture
by Yu Hui-chan and Han Fu-ru, trans. by Shuai Xue-zhong
ISBN 0-936185-78-3
ISBN 978-0-936185-78-1

A HANDBOOK OF CHINESE HEMATOLOGY
by Simon Becker
ISBN 1-891845-16-0
ISBN 978-1-891845-16-1

A HANDBOOK OF TCM PATTERNS
& THEIR TREATMENTS   Second Edition
by Bob Flaws & Daniel Finney
ISBN 0-936185-70-8
ISBN 978-0-936185-70-5

A HANDBOOK OF TRADITIONAL
CHINESE DERMATOLOGY
by Liang Jian-hui, trans. by Zhang Ting-liang
& Bob Flaws
ISBN 0-936185-46-5
ISBN 978-0-936185-46-0

A HANDBOOK OF TRADITIONAL
CHINESE GYNECOLOGY
by Zhejiang College of TCM, trans. by Zhang Ting-liang
& Bob Flaws
ISBN 0-936185-06-6 (4th edit.)
ISBN 978-0-936185-06-4

A HANDBOOK of TCM PEDIATRICS
by Bob Flaws
ISBN 0-936185-72-4
ISBN 978-0-936185-72-9

THE HEART & ESSENCE OF DAN-XI'S
METHODS OF TREATMENT
by Xu Dan-xi, trans. by Yang Shou-zhong
ISBN 0-926185-50-3
ISBN 978-0-936185-50-7

HERB TOXICITIES & DRUG INTERACTIONS:
A Formula Approach
by Fred Jennes with Bob Flaws
ISBN 1-891845-26-8
ISBN 978-1-891845-26-0

IMPERIAL SECRETS OF HEALTH & LONGEVITY
by Bob Flaws
ISBN 0-936185-51-1
ISBN 978-0-936185-51-4

INSIGHTS OF A SENIOR ACUPUNCTURIST
by Miriam Lee
ISBN 0-936185-33-3
ISBN 978-0-936185-33-0

INTEGRATED PHARMACOLOGY: Combining Modern
Pharmacology with Chinese Medicine
by Dr. Greg Sperber with Bob Flaws
ISBN 1-891845-41-1
ISBN 978-0-936185-41-3

INTRODUCTION TO THE USE OF
PROCESSED CHINESE MEDICINALS
by Philippe Sionneau
ISBN 0-936185-62-7
ISBN 978-0-936185-62-0

KEEPING YOUR CHILD HEALTHY WITH
CHINESE MEDICINE
by Bob Flaws
ISBN 0-936185-71-6
ISBN 978-0-936185-71-2

THE LAKESIDE MASTER'S STUDY OF THE PULSE
by Li Shi-zhen, trans. by Bob Flaws
ISBN 1-891845-01-2
ISBN 978-1-891845-01-7

MANAGING MENOPAUSE NATURALLY WITH
CHINESE MEDICINE
by Honora Lee Wolfe
ISBN 0-936185-98-8
ISBN 978-0-936185-98-9

MASTER HUA'S CLASSIC OF THE CENTRAL
VISCERA
by Hua Tuo, trans. by Yang Shou-zhong
ISBN 0-936185-43-0
ISBN 978-0-936185-43-9

THE MEDICAL I CHING: Oracle of the Healer Within
by Miki Shima
ISBN 0-936185-38-4
ISBN 978-0-936185-38-5

MENOPAIUSE & CHINESE MEDICINE
by Bob Flaws
ISBN 1-891845-40-3
ISBN 978-1-891845-40-6

MOXIBUSTION: A MODERN CLINICAL HANDBOOK
by Lorraine Wilcox
ISBN 1-891845-49-7
ISBN 978-1-891845-49-9

MOXIBUSTION: THE POWER OF MUGWORT FIRE
by Lorraine Wilcox
ISBN 1-891845-46-2
ISBN 978-1-891845-46-8

A NEW AMERICAN ACUPUNTURE By Mark Seem
ISBN 0-936185-44-9
ISBN 978-0-936185-44-6

POCKET ATLAS OF CHINESE MEDICINE
Edited by Marne and Kevin Ergil
ISBN 3-131416-11-7
ISBN 978-3-131416-11-7

POINTS FOR PROFIT: The Essential Guide to Practice
Success for Acupuncturists 4rd Edition
by Honora Wolfe, Eric Strand & Marilyn Allen
ISBN 1-891845-25-X
ISBN 978-1-891845-25-3

PRINCIPLES OF CHINESE MEDICAL ANDROLOGY:
An Integrated Approach to Male Reproductive and
Urological Health by Bob Damone
ISBN 1-891845-45-4
ISBN 978-1-891845-45-1

PRINCE WEN HUI's COOK: Chinese Dietary Therapy
By Bob Flaws & Honora Wolfe
ISBN 0-912111-05-4
ISBN 978-0-912111-05-6

THE PULSE CLASSIC:
A Translation of the Mai Jing
by Wang Shu-he, trans. by Yang Shou-zhong
ISBN 0-936185-75-9
ISBN 978-0-936185-75-0

THE SECRET OF CHINESE PULSE DIAGNOSIS
by Bob Flaws
ISBN 0-936185-67-8
ISBN 978-0-936185-67-5

SECRET SHAOLIN FORMULAS FOR THE
TREATMENT OF EXTERNAL INJURY
by De Chan, trans. by Zhang Ting-liang & Bob Flaws
ISBN 0-936185-08-2
ISBN 978-0-936185-08-8

STATEMENTS OF FACT IN TRADITIONAL
CHINESE MEDICINE   Revised & Expanded
by Bob Flaws
ISBN 0-936185-52-X
ISBN 978-0-936185-52-1

STICKING TO THE POINT: A Step-by-Step Approach
to TCM Acupuncture Therapy
by Bob Flaws & Honora Wolfe   2 Condensed Books
ISBN 1-891845-47-0
ISBN 978-1-891845-47-5

A STUDY OF DAOIST ACUPUNCTURE
by Liu Zheng-cai
ISBN 1-891845-08-X
ISBN 978-1-891845-08-6

THE SUCCESSFUL CHINESE HERBALIST
by Bob Flaws and Honora Lee Wolfe
ISBN 1-891845-29-2
ISBN 978-1-891845-29-1

THE SYSTEMATIC CLASSIC OF ACUPUNCTURE &
MOXIBUSTION
A translation of the Jia Yi Jing
by Huang-fu Mi, trans. by Yang Shou-zhong & Charles Chace
ISBN 0-936185-29-5
ISBN 978-0-936185-29-3

THE TAO OF HEALTHY EATING: DIETARY
WISDOM ACCORDING TO CHINESE MEDICINE
by Bob Flaws   Second Edition
ISBN 0-936185-92-9
ISBN 978-0-936185-92-7

TEACH YOURSELF TO READ MODERN
MEDICAL CHINESE
by Bob Flaws
ISBN 0-936185-99-6
ISBN 978-0-936185-99-6

TEST PREP WORKBOOK FOR BASIC TCM THEORY
by Zhong Bai-song
ISBN 1-891845-43-8
ISBN 978-1-891845-43-7

TEST PREP WORKBOOK FOR THE NCCAOM BIO-
MEDICINE MODULE: Exam Preparation & Study Guide
by Zhong Bai-song
ISBN 1-891845-34-9
ISBN 978-1-891845-34-5

TREATING PEDIATRIC BED-WETTING WITH
ACUPUNCTURE & CHINESE MEDICINE
by Robert Helmer
ISBN 1-891845-33-0
ISBN 978-1-891845-33-8

TREATISE on the SPLEEN & STOMACH: A
Translation and annotation of Li Dong-yuan's
Pi Wei Lun
by Bob Flaws
ISBN 0-936185-41-4
ISBN 978-0-936185-41-5

THE TREATMENT OF CARDIOVASCULAR DIS-
EASES WITH CHINESE MEDICINE
by Simon Becker, Bob Flaws &
Robert Casañas, MD
ISBN 1-891845-27-6
ISBN 978-1-891845-27-7

THE TREATMENT OF DIABETES MELLITUS WITH
CHINESE MEDICINE
by Bob Flaws, Lynn Kuchinski &
Robert Casañas, M.D.
ISBN 1-891845-21-7
ISBN 978-1-891845-21-5

THE TREATMENT OF DISEASE IN TCM, Vol. 1:
Diseases of the Head & Face, Including Mental &
Emotional Disorders   New Edition
by Philippe Sionneau & Lü Gang
ISBN 0-936185-69-4
ISBN 978-0-936185-69-9

THE TREATMENT OF DISEASE IN TCM, Vol. II:
Diseases of the Eyes, Ears, Nose, & Throat
by Sionneau & Lü
ISBN 0-936185-73-2
ISBN 978-0-936185-73-6

THE TREATMENT OF DISEASE IN TCM, Vol. III:
Diseases of the Mouth, Lips, Tongue, Teeth & Gums
by Sionneau & Lü
ISBN 0-936185-79-1
ISBN 978-0-936185-79-8

THE TREATMENT OF DISEASE IN TCM, Vol IV:
Diseases of the Neck, Shoulders, Back, & Limbs
by Philippe Sionneau & Lü Gang
ISBN 0-936185-89-9
ISBN 978-0-936185-89-7

THE TREATMENT OF DISEASE IN TCM, Vol V:
Diseases of the Chest & Abdomen
by Philippe Sionneau & Lü Gang
ISBN 1-891845-02-0
ISBN 978-1-891845-02-4

THE TREATMENT OF DISEASE IN TCM, Vol VI:
Diseases of the Urogential System & Proctology
by Philippe Sionneau & Lü Gang
ISBN 1-891845-05-5
ISBN 978-1-891845-05-5

THE TREATMENT OF DISEASE IN TCM, Vol VII:
General Symptoms
by Philippe Sionneau & Lü Gang
ISBN 1-891845-14-4
ISBN 978-1-891845-14-7

THE TREATMENT OF EXTERNAL DISEASES WITH
ACUPUNCTURE & MOXIBUSTION
by Yan Cui-lan and Zhu Yun-long, trans. by Yang Shou-zhong
ISBN 0-936185-80-5
ISBN 978-0-936185-80-4

THE TREATMENT OF MODERN WESTERN
MEDICAL DISEASES WITH CHINESE MEDICINE
by Bob Flaws & Philippe Sionneau
ISBN 1-891845-20-9
ISBN 978-1-891845-20-8

UNDERSTANDING THE DIFFICULT PATIENT: A
Guide for Practitioners of Oriental Medicine
by Nancy Bilello, RN, L.ac.
ISBN 1-891845-32-2
ISBN 978-1-891845-32-1

WESTERN PHYSICAL EXAM SKILLS FOR
PRACTITIONERS OF ASIAN MEDICINE
by Bruce H. Robinson & Honora Lee Wolfe
ISBN 1-891845-48-9
ISBN 978-1-891845-48-2

YI LIN GAI CUO (Correcting the Errors in the Forest of
Medicine)
by Wang Qing-ren
ISBN 1-891845-39-X
ISBN 978-1-891845-39-0

70 ESSENTIAL CHINESE HERBAL FORMULAS
by Bob Flaws
ISBN 0-936185-59-7
ISBN 978-0-936185-59-0

160 ESSENTIAL CHINESE READY-MADE
MEDICINES
by Bob Flaws
ISBN 1-891945-12-8
ISBN 978-1-891945-12-3

630 QUESTIONS & ANSWERS ABOUT CHINESE
HERBAL MEDICINE:
A Workbook & Study Guide
by Bob Flaws
ISBN 1-891845-04-7
ISBN 978-1-891845-04-8

260 ESSENTIAL CHINESE MEDICINALS
by Bob Flaws
ISBN 1-891845-03-9
ISBN 978-1-891845-03-1

750 QUESTIONS & ANSWERS ABOUT
ACUPUNCTURE
Exam Preparation & Study Guide
by Fred Jennes
ISBN 1-891845-22-5
ISBN 978-1-891845-22-2